LOW LECTIN FOODS

By

Calvin M. Duncan

All rights reserved. No part of this publication may be reproduced, distributed, or transmitted in any form or by any means, including photocopying, recording or other electronic or mechanical methods, without the prior written permission of the publisher, except in the case of brief quotation embodied in critical reviews and certain other noncommercial uses permitted by copyright law

Copyright by Calvin M. Duncan 2023

Table of Contents

Figs

Garlic

Ginger

Grapes

Green beans

Kale

Kiwi

Leeks

Lemons

Lettuce

Macadamia nuts

Mangoes

Mushrooms

Nectarines

Okra

Onions

Oranges

Papaya

Peaches

Pears

Peppers (bell peppers, chili peppers)

Pineapple

Plums

Pomegranates

Radishes

Raspberries

Spinach

Squash (butternut, acorn)

Sweet potatoes

Tomatoes

Watercress

Watermelon

Zucchini

Introduction

Lectins are a class of proteins that are widely distributed in nature, found in various plants, animals, and microorganisms. They play a crucial role in biological processes, particularly in the context of cell communication, immune system modulation, and plant defense mechanisms. While lectins have diverse functions, their potential impact on human health has been a subject of interest and debate.

In plants, lectins serve as defense mechanisms by binding to carbohydrates on the surface of pathogens, such as bacteria and fungi, preventing their invasion. In addition to their role in defense, lectins also contribute to the plant's ability to fix nitrogen and interact with symbiotic bacteria. However, some lectins can be toxic and harmful if consumed in large quantities, particularly those found in certain raw or undercooked legumes and grains.

The potential concern with lectins in the human diet arises from their ability to bind to carbohydrates present on the surface of cells. When consumed, lectins can interact with cells in the human body, leading to a range of effects. One notable aspect is their interaction with the lining of the digestive tract. Lectins may bind to the cells of the gut lining, disrupting the integrity of the mucosal barrier. This has led to the hypothesis that lectins could contribute to conditions like leaky gut syndrome, where there is an increased permeability of the intestinal wall.

Proponents of a low-lectin diet argue that reducing the intake of certain high-lectin foods may help mitigate potential adverse effects associated with lectins. Foods that are commonly recommended to be limited in a low-lectin diet include legumes (such as beans, lentils, and peanuts), grains (especially those containing gluten), nightshade vegetables (like tomatoes, peppers, and eggplants), and certain seeds. It is important to note that cooking can often reduce lectin content in foods, so properly preparing these items can mitigate some of the concerns.

Supporters of the low-lectin diet suggest that it may be particularly beneficial for individuals with autoimmune conditions or digestive issues, as lectins have been implicated in inflammatory responses and immune system activation. However, it's crucial to recognize that the scientific evidence supporting the widespread adoption of a low-lectin diet is limited and not without controversy.

Furthermore, many foods containing lectins also offer essential nutrients, fiber, and other bioactive compounds that contribute to overall health. Completely avoiding lectins might result in the exclusion of nutrient-rich foods from the diet, potentially leading to nutritional deficiencies.

In conclusion, lectins are a diverse group of proteins with important roles in biological processes, particularly in plants. While concerns about their potential impact on human health exist, the evidence supporting the need for a widespread low-lectin diet is not conclusive. For individuals considering such a dietary approach, it is advisable to consult with a healthcare professional or a

registered dietitian to ensure a balanced and nutrient-rich diet while addressing specific health concerns.

Guide to use these foods

Adopting a low lectin foods approach involves a mindful and purposeful selection of dietary options to potentially support overall health and well-being. This comprehensive guide explores the practical aspects of incorporating low lectin foods into your daily life, providing a roadmap for making informed choices and embracing a sustainable and balanced lifestyle.

Understanding the Foundations of Low Lectin Foods:

Before delving into the practical aspects, it's crucial to have a clear understanding of what low lectin foods entail. Lectins are proteins found in various foods, and while some are beneficial, others can potentially have adverse effects on human health, particularly in relation to digestion and inflammation. Low lectin foods, therefore, are those that contain lower levels of these proteins, and their inclusion in your diet can be a strategic step toward optimizing your nutritional intake.

Building Awareness of High Lectin Foods:

The first practical step in utilizing low lectin foods is to identify and limit the consumption of high lectin foods. Legumes, grains, nightshade vegetables, and certain seeds are common culprits. Recognizing these sources allows you to make intentional choices when planning your meals and snacks. While the idea is not necessarily to eliminate these foods entirely, being mindful of their lectin content helps in managing your overall dietary intake.

Exploring Low Lectin Alternatives:

The cornerstone of a successful low lectin diet lies in diversifying your food choices with alternatives that are naturally low in lectins. Vegetables like leafy greens, broccoli, and cauliflower, along with proteins from pasture-raised meats, poultry, and wild-caught fish, form

the basis of a lectin-conscious diet. Additionally, incorporating healthy fats from sources like avocados, olive oil, and nuts further enhances the nutritional profile of your meals.

Mastering Cooking Techniques to Reduce Lectins:

Cooking methods play a pivotal role in mitigating lectin content in foods. Soaking, fermenting, and proper cooking are effective techniques to reduce lectin levels. For example, soaking and cooking legumes thoroughly can enhance their digestibility, while fermenting grains before cooking may break down lectins. Adopting these cooking practices allows you to enjoy a diverse range of foods while minimizing potential lectin-related concerns.

Mindful Meal Planning:

Practical integration of low lectin foods involves thoughtful meal planning. Create a weekly meal plan that incorporates a balance of proteins, healthy fats, and a variety of low lectin vegetables. This not only streamlines your grocery shopping but also ensures that you have a well-rounded and lectin-conscious assortment of foods readily available. Consider experimenting with new recipes to keep your meals interesting and satisfying.

Snacking Strategies for Success:

Snacking is an integral part of daily life, and on a low lectin diet, it's essential to choose snacks that align with your goals. Nut butter on celery sticks, sliced cucumber with guacamole, or a handful of nuts are examples of satisfying and low lectin snack options. Being mindful of your snacking choices contributes to the overall success of your dietary journey.

Navigating Social Situations:

Eating out or attending social gatherings may pose challenges, but with strategic planning, you can navigate these situations successfully. Communicate your dietary needs to hosts, choose restaurants with options that align with your goals, and focus on lean proteins, salads, and non-nightshade vegetables when dining out. Making special requests when necessary ensures that your dietary preferences are accommodated without compromising social engagements.

Embracing Diversity in Your Diet:

While the primary focus is on reducing lectin intake, it's equally important to maintain a diverse and well-rounded diet. Excluding entire food groups may lead to nutritional deficiencies. Ensure

your low lectin diet includes a variety of vegetables, fruits, proteins, and fats to provide essential nutrients for overall health. Embracing diversity in your diet not only enhances nutritional value but also contributes to a more enjoyable and sustainable approach.

Listening to Your Body:

As you embark on your low lectin journey, pay close attention to how your body responds. Individual tolerance to lectins varies, and factors such as gut health, genetics, and overall well-being play a role. If you experience digestive discomfort or notice changes in your health, consider adjusting your food choices or consulting with a healthcare professional for personalized advice.

Staying Informed and Adapting:

Nutritional science is dynamic, and staying informed about the latest research is essential. Keep abreast of updates related to lectins and dietary health, allowing you to make informed decisions based on new information. Being adaptable enables you to tailor your low lectin diet to suit your changing needs, ensuring that your approach remains relevant and effective.

Seeking Professional Guidance:

While this guide provides practical advice, it's essential to recognize the individuality of dietary needs. Consulting with a healthcare professional or a registered dietitian offers personalized guidance based on your health goals, medical history, and lifestyle. They can help you create a sustainable low lectin diet that aligns with your unique needs, ensuring overall well-being and long-term success.

In conclusion, incorporating low lectin foods into your daily life involves a thoughtful and intentional approach to nutrition. By understanding the foundations of low lectin foods, building awareness of high lectin sources, exploring alternatives, mastering cooking techniques, and adopting mindful meal planning and snacking strategies, you can create a sustainable and enjoyable low lectin lifestyle. Embracing diversity in your diet, listening to your body, staying informed, and seeking professional guidance contribute to a holistic and personalized approach to optimizing your health through low lectin nutrition.

Almonds

Almonds, often referred to as the "king of nuts," are not just a delicious snack; they are a nutritional powerhouse with a rich history dating back thousands of years. Originating from the Middle East and South Asia, almonds have become a globally celebrated food, cherished for their delicate flavor, versatility, and an impressive array of health benefits.

Nutritional Profile: Almonds boast a remarkable nutritional composition, making them a valuable addition to a balanced diet. A 1-ounce (28-gram) serving of almonds provides approximately:

- Calories: 160

- Protein: 6 grams

- Fat: 14 grams (of which 9 grams are monounsaturated fat)

- Carbohydrates: 6 grams (of which 3.5 grams are dietary fiber)

- Vitamin E: 7.3 mg (37% of the Recommended Daily Allowance, RDA)

- Magnesium: 76 mg (19% of the RDA)

Heart Health: One of the standout features of almonds is their heart-healthy profile. The monounsaturated fats, along with polyunsaturated fats and low saturated fat content, contribute to improving cholesterol levels. Regular almond consumption has been associated with a reduced risk of heart disease.

Weight Management: Contrary to conventional wisdom associating nuts with weight gain, almonds have been linked to weight management. The combination of protein, healthy fats, and fiber in almonds induces a feeling of fullness, potentially leading to reduced overall calorie intake.

Blood Sugar Control: Almonds have a low glycemic index, meaning they cause a gradual rise in blood sugar levels. The fiber content aids in slowing down glucose absorption, making them a suitable choice for individuals managing diabetes or those looking to stabilize blood sugar levels.

Nutrient-Rich Antioxidants: Almonds are a rich source of antioxidants, including vitamin E, which helps protect cells from oxidative damage. Antioxidants play a crucial role in reducing inflammation and supporting overall health.

Bone Health: The mineral duo of magnesium and phosphorus in almonds contributes to maintaining strong and healthy bones. Adequate magnesium intake is essential for bone density and overall skeletal health.

Skin Health: Vitamin E, present abundantly in almonds, is renowned for its skin-nourishing properties. Regular consumption may contribute to maintaining healthy skin and protecting against sun damage.

Culinary Versatility: Almonds are incredibly versatile in the kitchen. They can be enjoyed in various forms:

- Raw Almonds: A convenient and nutritious snack.

- Almond Butter: A creamy and delicious spread.

- Almond Milk: A popular dairy milk alternative.

- Almond Flour: Used in gluten-free baking.

- Sliced or Chopped Almonds: Perfect for adding crunch to salads, yogurt, or desserts.

Sustainability: Almond trees have a unique ecological benefit. They are pollinated by honeybees, contributing to the well-being of these crucial pollinators. However, almond cultivation has faced scrutiny due to water usage concerns, particularly in regions with water scarcity.

Considerations: While almonds offer a myriad of health benefits, moderation is key. Almonds are energy-dense, so excessive consumption may lead to an increase in calorie intake. Additionally, individuals with nut allergies should exercise caution, and it's advisable to choose unsalted and unflavored varieties to avoid unnecessary sodium and sugars.

Conclusion:

Almonds, with their delectable taste and unparalleled nutritional benefits, have rightfully earned their place as a superfood. Whether enjoyed on their own, sprinkled on salads, or blended into a creamy butter, almonds are a delightful addition to a health-conscious diet. As science continues to uncover their numerous health advantages, almonds remain a timeless and wholesome snack, embodying the essence of nature's gifts to our well-being.

Apples

Apples, the quintessential fruit, have been a symbol of health and vitality for centuries. With a history deeply rooted in various cultures, apples are not only a delicious snack but also a nutritional powerhouse. From their crispy texture to their versatile uses in culinary endeavors, apples offer a multitude of benefits that make them a staple in diets around the world.

Nutritional Bounty: Apples are low in calories but high in essential nutrients, making them an ideal choice for those seeking a healthy and satisfying snack. A medium-sized apple (about 182 grams) contains approximately:

- Calories: 95

- Fiber: 4 grams

- Vitamin C: 14% of the Recommended Daily Allowance (RDA)

- Potassium: 6% of the RDA

- Vitamin K: 5% of the RDA

Dietary Fiber for Digestive Health: One of the most significant contributions of apples to health is their fiber content. Apples contain both soluble and insoluble fiber, aiding digestion and promoting gut health. The soluble fiber, specifically pectin, is known for its cholesterol-lowering effects and its potential role in stabilizing blood sugar levels.

Antioxidant Richness: Apples are a rich source of antioxidants, including flavonoids and polyphenols. These compounds play a crucial role in combating oxidative stress, reducing inflammation, and protecting cells from damage caused by free radicals.

Heart Health Support: Regular apple consumption has been linked to a lower risk of heart disease. The soluble fiber in apples helps lower blood cholesterol levels, and the potassium content may contribute to maintaining healthy blood pressure.

Blood Sugar Regulation: Despite their natural sweetness, apples have a low glycemic index, meaning they cause a gradual rise in blood sugar levels. This makes them a suitable choice for individuals managing diabetes or those looking to regulate blood sugar levels.

Hydration and Oral Health: Apples have a high water content, contributing to hydration. Additionally, their natural crispiness can help stimulate saliva production, promoting oral health by reducing the risk of tooth decay.

Weight Management: Apples make for a satisfying and portable snack, making them a valuable ally in weight management. The combination of fiber and water content promotes a feeling of fullness, potentially reducing overall calorie intake.

Varieties and Culinary Uses: The sheer variety of apple cultivars offers an array of flavors, textures, and colors. From the sweetness of Honeycrisp to the tartness of Granny Smith, apples cater to diverse palates. Culinary uses are equally diverse:

  - Fresh Snacking: Enjoyed as a convenient and nutritious on-the-go snack.

  - Salads: Sliced apples add a sweet and crunchy element to both green and fruit salads.

  - Baking: A staple in pies, crisps, muffins, and cakes, apples lend their natural sweetness and moisture to a myriad of baked goods.

  - Sauces and Compotes: Cooked down into sauces or compotes, apples make a versatile accompaniment to both sweet and savory dishes.

Environmental Impact: Apples are relatively sustainable fruits. They grow in a variety of climates, reducing the environmental footprint associated with transportation. However, like many crops, apple cultivation may involve the use of pesticides, making it advisable to choose organic options when possible.

Considerations: While apples are a wholesome addition to most diets, some individuals may need to moderate their intake if they have sensitivities to fructose. Washing apples thoroughly or choosing organic options can help reduce pesticide exposure.

Conclusion:

Apples, with their satisfying crunch, natural sweetness, and impressive nutritional profile, truly embody the adage "an apple a day keeps the doctor away." Whether enjoyed fresh, baked into a pie, or sliced onto a salad, the versatility and health benefits of apples make them a timeless and delicious fruit that continues to capture the hearts and taste buds of people worldwide.

Apricots

Apricots, with their delicate golden hue and velvety texture, are a luscious and nutritious fruit that signals the arrival of summer. Native to Central Asia, apricots have been cultivated for thousands of years and are celebrated not only for their sweet taste but also for their myriad health benefits. From their rich vitamin and mineral content to their versatility in culinary applications, apricots bring a burst of sunshine to both our palates and nutritional profiles.

Nutritional Riches: Apricots are a nutrient-dense fruit, providing an array of essential vitamins and minerals in a delicious package. A standard serving of apricots (about four apricots or 100 grams) contains approximately:

- Calories: 48

- Vitamin A: 12% of the Recommended Daily Allowance (RDA)

- Vitamin C: 9% of the RDA

- Potassium: 3% of the RDA

- Fiber: 2 grams

Rich in Antioxidants: Apricots are loaded with antioxidants, including beta-carotene, which gives them their vibrant orange color. Antioxidants play a crucial role in neutralizing free radicals, protecting cells from damage, and supporting overall health.

Eye Health: The high concentration of beta-carotene in apricots contributes to eye health. Beta-carotene is converted into vitamin A in the body, playing a vital role in maintaining good vision and preventing age-related macular degeneration.

Heart Health: Apricots contain potassium, a mineral that helps regulate blood pressure and maintain cardiovascular health. The fiber content also contributes to heart health by helping to lower cholesterol levels.

Digestive Health: Apricots are a good source of dietary fiber, aiding in digestion and promoting a healthy gut. Fiber adds bulk to the stool and helps prevent constipation.

Natural Sweetness: Apricots offer a natural and satisfying sweetness, making them a healthier alternative to processed sweets. Their natural sugars, combined with fiber, provide a quick energy boost without causing rapid spikes in blood sugar levels.

Culinary Versatility: Apricots lend themselves to a variety of culinary applications, enhancing both sweet and savory dishes. Here are some ways to enjoy apricots in the kitchen:

- Fresh Snacking: Enjoyed on their own as a refreshing and portable snack.

- Desserts: A star ingredient in pies, tarts, jams, and preserves, apricots bring a sweet and tart flavor to a myriad of desserts.

- Salads: Sliced apricots add a burst of flavor to both green salads and grain-based salads.

- Sauces and Chutneys: Cooked down into sauces or chutneys, apricots make a delightful accompaniment to meats, cheeses, or desserts.

Seasonal Delight: Apricots are typically in season during the summer months, making them a delightful and anticipated addition to farmers' markets and grocery stores. Consuming fruits and vegetables in season often ensures optimal flavor and nutritional content.

Drying and Preservation: Dried apricots are a convenient way to enjoy this fruit year-round. However, it's essential to choose varieties without added sugars or sulfites to maximize health benefits.

Considerations: While apricots offer numerous health benefits, it's crucial to consume them in moderation. Excessive intake of any fruit, due to natural sugars, may contribute to calorie overconsumption. Additionally, individuals with known allergies to stone fruits should exercise caution.

Conclusion:

Apricots, with their sun-kissed glow and sweet-tart flavor, are a true emblem of summer's bounty. From their impressive nutrient profile to their culinary versatility, apricots offer a golden opportunity to savor the season's delights while nourishing the body. Whether enjoyed fresh, dried, or as part of a delectable recipe, apricots stand as golden gems, reminding us of the abundant and diverse gifts nature provides for our well-being.

Asparagus

Asparagus, with its slender and elegant spears, is a culinary delight that heralds the arrival of spring. This versatile vegetable not only graces our plates with its unique flavor and texture but also brings an impressive array of nutrients and health benefits. From its historical roots to its modern-day culinary applications, asparagus stands as a symbol of freshness, vitality, and culinary creativity.

A Nutrient-Rich Superfood: Asparagus is a nutritional powerhouse, offering a rich supply of essential vitamins and minerals. A standard serving (about 100 grams) provides approximately:

- Calories: 20

- Protein: 2.2 grams

- Fiber: 2.1 grams

- Vitamin K: 41% of the Recommended Daily Allowance (RDA)

- Vitamin C: 14% of the RDA

- Folate (Vitamin B9): 17% of the RDA

- Iron: 12% of the RDA

Rich in Antioxidants: Asparagus is a rich source of antioxidants, including vitamins A and C, which play a crucial role in neutralizing free radicals and supporting overall health. These antioxidants contribute to anti-inflammatory and anti-aging effects.

Digestive Health: Asparagus is a good source of dietary fiber, promoting digestive health by adding bulk to the stool and aiding in regular bowel movements. This fiber content also supports a healthy gut microbiome.

Heart Health: Asparagus contains folate, a B-vitamin that plays a role in cardiovascular health. Folate helps regulate homocysteine levels, and elevated homocysteine is associated with an increased risk of heart disease.

Low in Calories, High in Nutrients: Asparagus is a low-calorie vegetable, making it an excellent choice for those looking to manage their weight. Its nutrient density means you get a significant amount of vitamins and minerals for relatively few calories.

Culinary Versatility: Asparagus lends itself to a variety of culinary applications, adding a distinctive flavor and texture to dishes. Here are some popular ways to enjoy asparagus:

- Roasted or Grilled: Enhances the natural sweetness and imparts a delightful smokiness.

- Steamed: Preserves the crisp texture and vibrant color.

- In Salads: Adds a fresh and crunchy element to both warm and cold salads.

- In Stir-Fries: Complements a variety of vegetables and proteins.

- As a Side Dish: Whether sautéed, baked, or added to pasta dishes, asparagus elevates the overall meal.

Seasonal Delicacy: Asparagus is at its best during the spring season, and many enthusiasts eagerly anticipate its arrival at farmers' markets. Enjoying asparagus when it's in season often ensures optimal freshness and flavor.

Historical Significance: Asparagus has a long history, with records of its consumption dating back to ancient civilizations, including the Egyptians and Greeks. It was prized not only for its culinary qualities but also for its perceived medicinal benefits.

Considerations: While asparagus is a nutrient-rich vegetable, individuals with certain medical conditions, such as kidney issues, may need to moderate their asparagus intake due to its oxalate content. Asparagus can impart a distinct odor to urine in some people, a phenomenon linked to the presence of sulfur compounds in the vegetable.

Farm-to-Table Appeal: Given its relatively short growing season, asparagus often highlights the farm-to-table movement, emphasizing the importance of consuming fresh, locally sourced produce.

Conclusion:

Asparagus, with its slender beauty and nutritional prowess, is not just a vegetable; it's a symbol of the renewal and vibrancy that spring brings. Whether grilled, steamed, or tossed into a salad,

asparagus adds a touch of elegance to any dish while offering a host of health benefits. As we savor the crisp and flavorful spears, we celebrate not only the culinary joy but also the seasonal connection to nature's bounty that asparagus provides.

Avocado

Avocado, with its rich, buttery texture and distinctive flavor, has become a symbol of indulgence and health consciousness alike. This nutrient-dense fruit, native to Central and South America, has skyrocketed in popularity worldwide, thanks to its versatility, culinary appeal, and a remarkable array of health benefits. From its unique composition to its numerous culinary applications, avocados have earned their status as a beloved and sought-after superfood.

Nutrient-Rich Powerhouse: Avocados are densely packed with a variety of essential nutrients. A typical serving of avocado (about one cup or 150 grams) provides approximately:

- Calories: 240

- Healthy Fats: 21 grams (primarily monounsaturated fats)

- Protein: 3 grams

- Dietary Fiber: 13 grams

- Vitamin K: 26% of the Recommended Daily Allowance (RDA)

- Vitamin C: 17% of the RDA

- Vitamin E: 16% of the RDA

- Folate (Vitamin B9): 20% of the RDA

- Potassium: 708 mg (more than a banana)

Heart-Healthy Monounsaturated Fats: Avocados are rich in monounsaturated fats, particularly oleic acid. These heart-healthy fats have been associated with various cardiovascular benefits, including improved cholesterol levels and reduced inflammation.

High Fiber Content: The significant fiber content in avocados contributes to digestive health, aids in maintaining a healthy weight by promoting satiety, and helps regulate blood sugar levels.

Potassium for Blood Pressure Regulation: Avocados are an excellent source of potassium, a mineral crucial for maintaining proper blood pressure levels. Adequate potassium intake is associated with a lower risk of hypertension and stroke.

Antioxidant Protection: Avocados contain various antioxidants, including vitamin E and carotenoids. These compounds play a vital role in neutralizing free radicals, protecting cells from oxidative damage, and contributing to anti-aging effects.

Versatile Culinary Applications: Avocados have become a staple in various culinary creations, thanks to their creamy texture and mild taste. Here are some popular ways to enjoy avocados:

- Guacamole: Mashed avocados mixed with lime, cilantro, and other ingredients, making a classic dip.

- Avocado Toast: Sliced or mashed avocados on toasted bread, often topped with additional ingredients like poached eggs or tomatoes.

- Salads: Diced avocados add a creamy element to both green salads and grain bowls.

- Smoothies: Adding avocados to smoothies enhances the texture and provides a nutrient boost.

- Sandwiches and Wraps: Avocado slices or spreads bring a satisfying creaminess to sandwiches and wraps.

Skin Health and Beauty: The combination of healthy fats and antioxidants in avocados contributes to skin health. The monounsaturated fats may help maintain moisture, and antioxidants combat oxidative stress, potentially reducing signs of aging.

Sustainable and Eco-Friendly: Avocado trees thrive in diverse climates, and many avocado-producing regions prioritize sustainable farming practices. However, the high demand for avocados has raised concerns about deforestation in some areas, highlighting the importance of supporting sustainable sourcing.

Culinary Trends and Social Media Fame: Avocado has become a social media sensation, particularly through the viral trend of "avocado toast" and the sharing of aesthetically pleasing avocado-based dishes.

Considerations: While avocados offer numerous health benefits, their high caloric content means portion control is crucial, especially for those monitoring calorie intake. Additionally, individuals with latex allergies may experience cross-reactivity with avocados.

Conclusion:

Avocado, with its creamy allure and nutritional prowess, transcends its status as a mere fruit to become a culinary and dietary icon. Whether spread on toast, blended into a smoothie, or enjoyed in a salad, avocados bring a touch of indulgence to health-conscious eating. As we savor the

luxurious taste and reap the benefits of this green gem, avocados continue to be a delicious and nutritious cornerstone of modern, mindful living.

Bamboo Shoots

Bamboo shoots, the edible sprouts of bamboo plants, have been a culinary treasure in Asian cuisine for centuries. Harvested from various bamboo species, these young shoots offer a unique texture, subtle flavor, and a wealth of nutritional benefits. From traditional dishes to modern culinary innovations, bamboo shoots have made their mark as a versatile and healthy addition to a wide range of recipes.

Culinary Tradition: Bamboo shoots have been a staple in Asian cuisine for thousands of years, featuring prominently in dishes from China, Japan, Korea, and Southeast Asia. Their mild taste and ability to absorb flavors make them a versatile ingredient in both traditional and modern cooking.

Nutritional Profile: Bamboo shoots are low in calories but rich in nutrients. A 100-gram serving of bamboo shoots provides approximately:

- Calories: 27

- Protein: 2.6 grams

- Dietary Fiber: 2.2 grams

- Vitamin C: 5.6 milligrams (9% of the Recommended Daily Allowance, RDA)

- Vitamin B6: 0.2 milligrams (8% of the RDA)

- Minerals (Potassium, Phosphorus, and Magnesium): Contributing to overall health and electrolyte balance.

Rich in Antioxidants: Bamboo shoots contain antioxidants, including phenolic compounds, which help combat oxidative stress and inflammation in the body. Antioxidants play a crucial role in promoting overall health and reducing the risk of chronic diseases.

Digestive Health: The dietary fiber in bamboo shoots contributes to digestive health by promoting regular bowel movements and supporting a healthy gut microbiome. Fiber also helps control blood sugar levels and aids in weight management.

Low in Calories, High in Satisfaction: Bamboo shoots are an excellent choice for those looking to add bulk to their meals without significantly increasing calorie intake. Their satisfying texture and ability to absorb flavors make them a valuable ingredient in low-calorie and high-volume dishes.

Culinary Uses: Bamboo shoots are versatile in the kitchen and can be used in various culinary applications. Some popular dishes include:

- Stir-Fries: Added to stir-fries, bamboo shoots contribute a unique crunch and absorb the flavors of the dish.

- Soups: Commonly used in Asian soups, bamboo shoots add texture and enhance the overall taste.

- Curries: In Southeast Asian cuisine, bamboo shoots are a common ingredient in curries, providing a subtle flavor and tender texture.

- Spring Rolls: Bamboo shoots can be included in the filling of spring rolls, adding a delightful crunch.

Sustainability: Bamboo is a fast-growing and highly renewable resource. Harvesting bamboo shoots promotes sustainability as it encourages the growth of new shoots and does not harm the parent plant. This aligns with environmentally conscious practices in agriculture.

Caution in Consumption: While bamboo shoots are generally safe to eat, some varieties may contain compounds that need proper preparation before consumption. Bitter compounds, often found in certain types of bamboo shoots, can be removed through boiling or fermentation.

Cultural Significance: Bamboo has cultural significance in many Asian societies, symbolizing strength, resilience, and flexibility. The culinary use of bamboo shoots is deeply rooted in these cultural traditions.

Global Appeal: With the rise of global cuisine and increased interest in diverse flavors, bamboo shoots have found their way into kitchens worldwide. Their unique texture and ability to complement a variety of dishes make them a popular choice among chefs and home cooks alike.

Conclusion:

Bamboo shoots, with their delicate taste and versatile culinary applications, showcase the diversity and richness of Asian cuisine. From traditional dishes to modern interpretations, bamboo shoots continue to captivate food enthusiasts with their unique flavor, nutritional benefits, and cultural significance. As global palates embrace new and exciting tastes, bamboo shoots remain a crispy delicacy that bridges the past and present in the world of gastronomy.

Beets

Beets, with their striking deep red hue and earthy flavor, are a root vegetable that not only adds color to dishes but also brings a wealth of nutritional benefits. Known for their versatility in both culinary and health contexts, beets have been cultivated and consumed for centuries. From salads to soups, and juices to roasted dishes, beets have carved out a special place in diverse cuisines around the world.

Nutrient-Rich Powerhouse: Beets are loaded with essential nutrients that contribute to overall health and well-being. A one-cup serving of cooked beets (about 136 grams) provides approximately:

- Calories: 58

- Fiber: 3.8 grams

- Vitamin C: 6.7 milligrams (11% of the Recommended Daily Allowance, RDA)

- Folate (Vitamin B9): 148 micrograms (37% of the RDA)

- Potassium: 442 milligrams (13% of the RDA)

- Iron: 1.1 milligrams (6% of the RDA)

Rich in Antioxidants: Beets contain a unique set of antioxidants, including betalains, which contribute to their vibrant color. These antioxidants have been associated with anti-inflammatory and detoxification effects in the body, protecting cells from oxidative stress.

Heart Health: The nitrates in beets are converted into nitric oxide in the body, which can help dilate blood vessels, improve blood flow, and lower blood pressure. Regular beet consumption has been linked to cardiovascular benefits.

Digestive Health: Beets are an excellent source of dietary fiber, promoting digestive health by preventing constipation and supporting a healthy gut microbiome. The fiber content also contributes to a feeling of fullness, aiding in weight management.

Blood Sugar Regulation: The fiber in beets, combined with their low glycemic index, makes them a suitable food for individuals managing blood sugar levels. Beets may help stabilize glucose levels and reduce the risk of type 2 diabetes.

Culinary Versatility: Beets lend themselves to a variety of culinary applications, both raw and cooked. Some popular ways to enjoy beets include:

- Roasted: Enhances their natural sweetness and intensifies flavor.

- Salads: Shredded or cubed beets add color and texture to salads.

- Juices: Beets are often juiced, either on their own or as part of a blended concoction.

- Soups: A common ingredient in borscht, a traditional Eastern European soup.

- Pickled: Beets are pickled in various cuisines, offering a tangy and vibrant addition to meals.

Detoxification Benefits: The betalains in beets are believed to support the body's natural detoxification processes. They may help eliminate toxins and promote liver health.

Athletic Performance: Some studies suggest that the nitrates in beets may enhance athletic performance by improving oxygen utilization and increasing endurance. This has led to the popular use of beet juice as a pre-exercise supplement.

Edible Greens: Beet greens, the leafy tops of the plant, are also edible and highly nutritious. They contain vitamins A, C, and K, as well as minerals like iron and calcium. Beet greens can be sautéed, steamed, or added to salads.

Natural Dyes: The intense color of beets has been used historically as a natural dye for fabrics and even as a food coloring agent. The rich pigment can impart vibrant hues to a variety of dishes.

Conclusion:

Beets, with their vibrant color and nutritional richness, are a testament to the bountiful offerings of the earth. Beyond their culinary appeal, beets bring a host of health benefits, making them a valuable addition to a balanced and varied diet. Whether enjoyed roasted, pickled, juiced, or as part of a refreshing salad, beets continue to captivate taste buds and nourish bodies, embodying the essence of wholesome and delicious nutrition.

Berries

Berries, encompassing a delightful spectrum of colors and flavors, are not only delicious but also pack a nutritional punch that makes them stand out in the world of fruits. Blueberries, strawberries, and raspberries, among others, are celebrated for their vibrant hues, natural sweetness, and a treasure trove of antioxidants. From supporting heart health to boosting brain function, these berries are not just treats for the taste buds; they are miniature nutrient powerhouses that offer a myriad of health benefits.

Blueberries:

- Nutrient Profile: Blueberries are rich in vitamin C, vitamin K, manganese, and antioxidants such as anthocyanins.

- Brain Health: The antioxidants in blueberries may have cognitive benefits, potentially improving memory and cognitive function.

- Heart Health: Blueberries have been linked to lowering blood pressure and reducing the risk of heart disease.

Strawberries:

- Nutrient Profile: Strawberries are high in vitamin C, manganese, folate, and antioxidants like quercetin.

- Skin Health: The vitamin C and antioxidants in strawberries contribute to skin health, helping to combat oxidative stress and promote collagen production.

- Heart Health: Strawberries have been associated with improved heart health by reducing oxidative stress and inflammation.

Raspberries:

- Nutrient Profile: Raspberries provide vitamin C, manganese, fiber, and antioxidants, including quercetin and ellagic acid.

- Digestive Health: The high fiber content in raspberries promotes digestive health by supporting regular bowel movements.

- Anti-Inflammatory Effects: The antioxidants in raspberries may help reduce inflammation in the body.

Antioxidant Richness: Anthocyanins: Berries, especially blueberries and raspberries, are rich in anthocyanins, powerful antioxidants linked to various health benefits, including reduced inflammation and oxidative stress.

Heart Health: Blood Pressure Regulation: The presence of compounds like flavonoids in berries has been associated with improved blood pressure regulation, contributing to heart health.

- Cholesterol Management: Berries may help lower bad cholesterol (LDL) levels and raise good cholesterol (HDL) levels.

Weight Management: Low in Calories, High in Fiber: Berries are relatively low in calories but high in dietary fiber, promoting a feeling of fullness and aiding in weight management.

Cancer-Fighting Properties: Ellagic Acid: Some berries, including raspberries, contain ellagic acid, which has been studied for its potential anti-cancer properties by inhibiting the growth of cancer cells.

Blood Sugar Control: Fiber Content: The fiber in berries, combined with their natural sugars, helps regulate blood sugar levels, making them a suitable choice for individuals managing diabetes.

Culinary Versatility:

  - Fresh Consumption: Berries are a delightful snack when enjoyed fresh and can be easily incorporated into various dishes.

  - Smoothies: Berries add a burst of flavor and nutritional goodness to smoothies.

  - Desserts: From pies and tarts to parfaits and sorbets, berries enhance the sweetness and visual appeal of desserts.

Seasonal Variety: Local and Seasonal Availability: Berries are often available seasonally, with local varieties offering peak freshness and flavor during specific times of the year.

Conclusion:

Berries, with their enchanting colors and health-promoting properties, are more than just sweet treats—they are nutritional gems that contribute to overall well-being. Whether enjoyed fresh, blended into a smoothie, or added to various dishes, these berries add a burst of flavor, antioxidants, and essential nutrients to our diets. With each bite, berries exemplify the harmony of taste and health, making them a delicious and nutritious choice for individuals seeking to nourish their bodies with the goodness of nature.

Broccoli

Broccoli, with its vibrant green florets and earthy flavor, is a cruciferous vegetable that stands out not only for its culinary versatility but also for its impressive nutritional profile. From supporting immune health to providing a rich source of vitamins and minerals, broccoli has rightfully earned its place as a nutrient-dense powerhouse in the world of vegetables.

Nutrient-Rich Superfood:

Broccoli is a nutritional dynamo, offering an abundance of essential vitamins and minerals. A one-cup serving of cooked broccoli (about 156 grams) provides approximately:

- Calories: 55

- Protein: 3.7 grams

- Fiber: 5.1 grams

- Vitamin C: 135% of the Recommended Daily Allowance (RDA)

- Vitamin K: 116% of the RDA

- Folate (Vitamin B9): 14% of the RDA

- Potassium: 8% of the RDA

- Manganese: 10% of the RDA

Immune Support: Broccoli is a rich source of vitamin C, a powerful antioxidant that supports the immune system by protecting cells from damage and aiding in the production of collagen.

Cancer-Fighting Properties: Broccoli contains compounds, such as sulforaphane and indole-3-carbinol, that have been studied for their potential anti-cancer effects. These compounds may help inhibit the growth of cancer cells and promote detoxification.

Heart Health: The fiber, potassium, and antioxidants in broccoli contribute to heart health. The fiber helps lower cholesterol levels, potassium supports healthy blood pressure, and antioxidants combat oxidative stress.

Bone Health: Broccoli is a good source of vitamin K and calcium, essential for bone health. Vitamin K is crucial for proper calcium utilization and bone mineralization.

Digestive Health: The fiber content in broccoli aids in digestion, promotes regular bowel movements, and supports a healthy gut microbiome. This can contribute to digestive health and weight management.

Anti-Inflammatory Effects: Broccoli contains antioxidants and anti-inflammatory compounds that may help reduce inflammation in the body, contributing to overall health.

Culinary Versatility: Broccoli is a versatile vegetable that can be enjoyed in various culinary preparations. Some popular ways to incorporate broccoli into your diet include:

- Steamed or Boiled: Preserves its crisp texture and vibrant color.

- Roasted: Enhances the natural sweetness and imparts a delightful smokiness.

- Stir-Fried: Adds a crunchy element to stir-fries.

- Soups and Casseroles: Blends well with other ingredients in comforting dishes.

- Raw in Salads: Grated or chopped broccoli can add a fresh and nutritious crunch to salads.

Easy to Grow: Broccoli is a cool-season vegetable that can be relatively easy to grow in home gardens. Its adaptability makes it a popular choice for home gardeners looking to cultivate their own produce.

Considerations: While broccoli offers numerous health benefits, some individuals may experience digestive discomfort when consuming large amounts of cruciferous vegetables. Cooking broccoli can make it more digestible for some people.

Conclusion:

Broccoli, with its crisp texture and nutritional prowess, is more than just a side dish—it's a symbol of health and well-being. Whether enjoyed as a standalone vegetable or incorporated into a variety of recipes, broccoli provides a flavorful and nutrient-packed addition to our plates. As we savor its green goodness, we celebrate the simple yet profound impact that this cruciferous vegetable has on our overall health and vitality.

Brussels Sprouts

Brussels sprouts, often misunderstood and occasionally underrated, are miniature cruciferous vegetables that pack a punch in terms of both flavor and nutrition. Resembling mini cabbages, these green gems offer a unique taste that, when prepared correctly, can transform into a savory delight. Beyond their culinary appeal, Brussels sprouts boast an impressive array of nutrients that contribute to overall health and well-being.

Nutrient-Rich Powerhouses: Brussels sprouts are dense with essential vitamins, minerals, and fiber. A one-cup serving of cooked Brussels sprouts (about 156 grams) provides approximately:

- Calories: 56

- Protein: 3.4 grams

- Fiber: 4.1 grams

- Vitamin C: 124% of the Recommended Daily Allowance (RDA)

- Vitamin K: 274% of the RDA

- Vitamin A: 15% of the RDA

- Folate (Vitamin B9): 24% of the RDA

Rich in Antioxidants: Brussels sprouts are packed with antioxidants, including vitamin C, which plays a vital role in neutralizing free radicals, supporting the immune system, and promoting healthy skin.

Cruciferous Benefits: As part of the cruciferous vegetable family, Brussels sprouts contain compounds like glucosinolates, which have been associated with potential cancer-fighting properties. These compounds may support detoxification processes in the body.

Heart Health: The fiber, potassium, and folate content in Brussels sprouts contribute to cardiovascular health. Fiber helps manage cholesterol levels, potassium supports healthy blood pressure, and folate aids in reducing homocysteine levels, a risk factor for heart disease.

Vitamin K for Bone Health: The exceptionally high vitamin K content in Brussels sprouts plays a crucial role in bone health. Vitamin K is essential for proper calcium utilization and bone mineralization.

Digestive Health: Brussels sprouts are an excellent source of fiber, promoting digestive health by preventing constipation and supporting a healthy gut microbiome.

Low in Calories, High in Nutrients: Brussels sprouts are low in calories but nutrient-dense, making them an excellent choice for those looking to manage their weight while ensuring optimal nutrition.

Culinary Versatility: Brussels sprouts may have a reputation for being disliked by some, but when prepared with care, they can be a culinary delight. Here are some ways to enjoy Brussels sprouts:

- Roasted: Enhances their natural sweetness and imparts a delightful caramelization.

- Pan-Seared or Sauteed: Results in a crispy exterior and tender interior.

- Shredded in Salads: Adds a crunchy and nutritious element to salads.

- Grilled: Develops a smoky flavor and enhances their texture.

- In Casseroles or Stir-Fries: Blends well with other ingredients, adding a nutritional boost.

Seasonal Delicacy: Brussels sprouts are typically in season during the fall and winter months, making them a delightful addition to holiday feasts and winter menus.

Considerations: While Brussels sprouts offer numerous health benefits, some individuals may experience digestive discomfort due to their fiber content. Cooking methods, such as roasting or steaming, can enhance digestibility.

Conclusion:

Brussels sprouts, with their petite stature and nutritional richness, are a testament to the wonders of cruciferous vegetables. As we appreciate their vibrant green color and savor their unique flavor, we also embrace the multitude of health benefits these mini cabbages bring to our plates. Whether roasted to perfection, incorporated into salads, or added to hearty winter stews, Brussels sprouts offer a delicious and nutrient-packed addition to a balanced and wholesome diet.

Cabbage

Cabbage, a humble and often overlooked member of the cruciferous vegetable family, is a nutritional powerhouse that has been cultivated and consumed for centuries. With its tightly packed leaves and crisp texture, cabbage brings a subtle sweetness and a wealth of health benefits to a wide array of dishes. From coleslaw to stir-fries, this cruciferous marvel has earned its place in diverse cuisines around the world.

Nutrient-Rich Superfood: Cabbage is a low-calorie vegetable but is rich in essential nutrients. A one-cup serving of shredded cabbage (about 89 grams) provides approximately:

- Calories: 22

- Fiber: 2.2 grams

- Vitamin C: 36% of the Recommended Daily Allowance (RDA)

- Vitamin K: 57% of the RDA

- Folate (Vitamin B9): 5% of the RDA

- Manganese: 6% of the RDA

Antioxidant Richness: Cabbage is a good source of antioxidants, including vitamin C and polyphenols. These compounds help combat oxidative stress, reduce inflammation, and contribute to overall health.

Cancer-Fighting Properties: Compounds found in cabbage, such as glucosinolates, have been studied for their potential cancer-fighting properties. These compounds may help inhibit the growth of cancer cells and support detoxification.

Digestive Health: The fiber content in cabbage promotes digestive health by preventing constipation and supporting a healthy gut microbiome. It adds bulk to the stool and aids in regular bowel movements.

Weight Management: Cabbage is low in calories and high in fiber, making it a filling and satisfying addition to meals. Its crunchiness adds texture without adding excessive calories.

Heart Health: The fiber and antioxidants in cabbage contribute to heart health. Fiber helps manage cholesterol levels, and antioxidants combat oxidative stress, reducing the risk of cardiovascular diseases.

Vitamin K for Bone Health: Cabbage is an excellent source of vitamin K, which is essential for proper blood clotting and bone health. Adequate vitamin K intake contributes to bone mineralization and density.

Culinary Versatility: Cabbage's versatility in the kitchen makes it a staple in various cuisines worldwide. Some popular ways to enjoy cabbage include:

- Coleslaw: Shredded cabbage mixed with a tangy dressing, often served as a side dish.

- Stir-Fries: Cabbage adds crunch and absorbs flavors in stir-fried dishes.

- Sauerkraut: Fermented cabbage, known for its probiotic benefits and tangy flavor.

- Soups and Stews: Cabbage is a hearty addition to soups and stews, adding both flavor and nutrients.

- Stuffed Cabbage Rolls: Cabbage leaves are filled with a mixture of meat and rice, then cooked in a savory sauce.

Economical and Long Shelf Life: Cabbage is an economical vegetable with a relatively long shelf life, making it accessible and practical for various households. Properly stored, cabbage can last for several weeks.

Historical Significance: Cabbage has a rich history, dating back to ancient civilizations. It has been a dietary staple for centuries, appreciated for its nutritional value and versatility in cooking.

Conclusion:

Cabbage, with its unassuming appearance and wealth of nutrients, is a testament to the nutritional treasures found in everyday vegetables. As we incorporate cabbage into our meals, whether raw or cooked, we celebrate not only its culinary versatility but also the diverse health benefits it brings to our tables. From supporting digestion to contributing to heart health, cabbage stands as a testament to the profound impact that simple, wholesome foods can have on our well-being.

Cauliflower

Cauliflower, a member of the cruciferous vegetable family, has transformed from a humble kitchen staple to a versatile culinary chameleon that adapts to a myriad of dishes. With its neutral taste and unique texture, cauliflower has become a popular substitute for traditional starches and grains, offering a low-calorie, nutrient-dense alternative. From creamy mashed cauliflower to trendy cauliflower rice, this cruciferous gem brings both culinary creativity and health benefits to the table.

Nutrient-Rich Profile: Cauliflower is a nutritional powerhouse, providing essential vitamins and minerals. A one-cup serving of raw cauliflower (about 107 grams) offers approximately:

- Calories: 27

- Fiber: 2 grams

- Vitamin C: 77% of the Recommended Daily Allowance (RDA)

- Vitamin K: 20% of the RDA

- Folate (Vitamin B9): 14% of the RDA

-Vitamin B6: 11% of the RDA

Cruciferous Health Benefits: As a cruciferous vegetable, cauliflower contains glucosinolates, compounds with potential anti-cancer properties. These compounds may support detoxification and inhibit the growth of cancer cells.

Rich in Antioxidants: Cauliflower is rich in antioxidants, including vitamin C and manganese. These antioxidants play a crucial role in neutralizing free radicals and supporting overall health.

Weight Management: Cauliflower is low in calories and carbohydrates, making it an excellent choice for those focusing on weight management. Its high fiber content adds bulk to meals, promoting a feeling of fullness.

Versatile Culinary Applications: The neutral flavor and unique texture of cauliflower make it a versatile ingredient in various culinary creations. Some popular ways to enjoy cauliflower include:

- Cauliflower Rice: Finely grated cauliflower used as a low-carb substitute for rice.

- Cauliflower Mash: Creamy mashed cauliflower as a healthier alternative to mashed potatoes.

- Cauliflower Pizza Crust: A gluten-free crust made from cauliflower, offering a lighter option for pizza lovers.

- Roasted Cauliflower: Simple yet flavorful, roasted cauliflower enhances its natural sweetness and develops a satisfying crunch.

- Cauliflower Wings: Battered and baked or fried cauliflower florets, often served with dipping sauces.

Fiber for Digestive Health: The fiber content in cauliflower promotes digestive health by preventing constipation and supporting a healthy gut microbiome. It aids in regular bowel movements and contributes to overall digestive well-being.

Low-Carb Alternative: Cauliflower has gained popularity as a low-carb alternative in various dishes. It serves as a versatile substitute for higher-carb ingredients like rice, potatoes, and flour.

Bone Health: Cauliflower contributes to bone health due to its vitamin K content, which plays a crucial role in bone mineralization and blood clotting.

Dietary Inclusion: Cauliflower is suitable for various dietary preferences and restrictions, including low-carb, keto, gluten-free, and plant-based diets.

Trendy and Innovative: The rise of health-conscious eating has propelled cauliflower into the spotlight, leading to innovative culinary trends and a newfound appreciation for its adaptability in the kitchen.

Conclusion:

Cauliflower, with its understated appearance and remarkable versatility, has emerged as a culinary hero in the quest for healthier, creative cooking. As we explore the numerous ways to incorporate cauliflower into our meals, we not only savor its subtle taste and diverse textures but also embrace

its contribution to our overall well-being. From nutrient-rich sides to innovative substitutes, cauliflower proves that simplicity in appearance can coexist with complexity in flavor and nutritional value, making it a valuable addition to the modern kitchen.

Celery

Celery, with its crunchy texture and distinctive flavor, is a low-calorie vegetable that has found its way into a variety of dishes and snacks. While often enjoyed for its satisfying crunch and refreshing taste, celery also boasts an impressive nutrient profile. From promoting hydration to contributing to digestive health, celery stands out as a versatile and healthful addition to a balanced diet.

Hydration and Low-Calorie Goodness: Celery is composed mostly of water, making it an excellent choice for hydration. With only about 10 calories per cup (about 101 grams), celery is a low-calorie snack that can be enjoyed guilt-free.

Nutrient Profile: Although low in calories, celery is not lacking in essential nutrients. A one-cup serving of chopped celery provides approximately:

- Calories: 16

- Dietary Fiber: 1.6 grams

- Vitamin K: 32% of the Recommended Daily Allowance (RDA)

- Vitamin A: 9% of the RDA

- Folate (Vitamin B9): 9% of the RDA

- Potassium: 8% of the RDA

Antioxidant Properties: Celery contains antioxidants, including flavonoids and polyphenols, which help combat oxidative stress and inflammation in the body. These compounds contribute to overall health and may play a role in disease prevention.

Hydration Support: The high water content in celery (about 95%) makes it a hydrating snack, promoting fluid balance in the body. Staying adequately hydrated is essential for various bodily functions, including digestion and temperature regulation.

Digestive Health: Celery is a good source of dietary fiber, aiding in digestion and promoting regular bowel movements. The fiber content contributes to a feeling of fullness, making it a satisfying and healthy snack option.

Blood Pressure Regulation: Celery contains compounds, such as phthalides, that may help lower blood pressure by relaxing blood vessel walls and improving blood flow. Including celery in a balanced diet may contribute to cardiovascular health.

Natural Diuretic: Celery has natural diuretic properties, promoting urine production and helping to flush out excess fluid from the body. This can be beneficial for individuals dealing with water retention.

Culinary Versatility: Celery is a versatile vegetable that can be enjoyed in various ways. It adds a refreshing crunch to:

- Snack Trays: Paired with dips or spreads.

- Salads: Providing a crisp texture and mild flavor.

- Soups and Stews: Enhancing both flavor and nutritional content.

- Smoothies: Adding a hydrating element to beverages.

Historical Significance: Celery has a long history of use, dating back to ancient times. It was prized by the ancient Greeks and Romans for its medicinal properties, and it has remained a staple in culinary traditions across cultures.

Considerations: While celery is generally well-tolerated, some individuals may be allergic to certain proteins in celery. Additionally, celery is part of the "Dirty Dozen," a list of produce items that may have higher pesticide residues, so choosing organic celery when possible may be advisable.

Conclusion:

Celery, with its crispness and nutritional virtues, transcends its role as a mere snack or salad component. Whether enjoyed for its hydrating qualities or appreciated for its contribution to digestive health, celery stands as a testament to the simple yet impactful role that vegetables play in our overall well-being. As we munch on its refreshing stalks, we not only enjoy a satisfying

crunch but also partake in a tradition that spans centuries, connecting us to the enduring and wholesome nature of this versatile vegetable.

Cherries

Cherries, with their vibrant colors and succulent flavors, are more than just a delightful summer treat. Whether enjoyed fresh, dried, or incorporated into various culinary creations, cherries are not only delicious but also pack a punch of nutrients and health benefits. From supporting heart health to reducing inflammation, these little gems contribute both taste and wellness to our plates.

Nutrient-Rich Goodness: Cherries are a nutrient-dense fruit, providing an array of vitamins, minerals, and antioxidants. A one-cup serving of pitted cherries (about 138 grams) offers approximately:

- Calories: 87

- Vitamin C: 16% of the Recommended Daily Allowance (RDA)

- Potassium: 10% of the RDA

- Dietary Fiber: 3 grams

- Anthocyanins: Powerful antioxidants responsible for the deep red and purple colors of cherries.

Antioxidant Powerhouse: Cherries, especially tart cherries, are rich in antioxidants, including anthocyanins and quercetin. These compounds have been associated with reducing oxidative stress and inflammation in the body.

Heart Health: The potassium content in cherries supports heart health by helping regulate blood pressure. Additionally, the anthocyanins in cherries may contribute to improved cardiovascular function.

Anti-Inflammatory Effects: Cherries have been studied for their potential to reduce inflammation and alleviate symptoms of inflammatory conditions, such as arthritis and gout. This anti-inflammatory property is attributed to the presence of anthocyanins and other bioactive compounds.

Melatonin for Sleep: Cherries, particularly tart cherries, are a natural source of melatonin, a hormone that regulates sleep-wake cycles. Consuming cherries or tart cherry juice may contribute to improved sleep quality and duration.

Joint Health: The anti-inflammatory properties of cherries may benefit joint health, potentially reducing pain and stiffness associated with conditions like osteoarthritis and gout.

Fiber for Digestive Health: Cherries contribute to digestive health due to their fiber content. Dietary fiber aids in regular bowel movements, promotes a healthy gut microbiome, and contributes to overall digestive well-being.

Culinary Versatility: Cherries lend themselves to a variety of culinary applications, adding sweetness and depth of flavor to both sweet and savory dishes. Some popular ways to enjoy cherries include:

- Fresh: Enjoyed as a snack or added to fruit salads.

- Dried: A convenient and portable option for snacking.

- Juices and Smoothies: Blended into refreshing beverages.

- Desserts: Used in pies, tarts, and cobblers.

- Savory Dishes: Paired with meats or incorporated into sauces for a sweet contrast.

Seasonal Delight: Cherries are often associated with the summer season, where their peak freshness and availability make them a highly anticipated and celebrated fruit.

Variety of Types: There are various types of cherries, including sweet cherries (like Bing and Rainier) and tart cherries (Montmorency). Each variety has its unique flavor profile, sweetness level, and culinary uses.

Conclusion:

Cherries, with their delectable taste and impressive nutritional profile, exemplify the marriage of flavor and health in the world of fruits. As we enjoy these juicy orbs, we not only savor their sweetness but also partake in the wholesome goodness they bring to our bodies. Cherries, in their myriad forms and varieties, stand as a reminder of the delightful and nourishing treasures found in nature's bounty.

Coconut

Coconut, often associated with tropical paradises, is not just a symbol of exotic locales but also a nutritional powerhouse with a myriad of uses. From its refreshing water to the versatile flesh and rich oil, the coconut palm provides a bounty of essential nutrients and culinary delights. Let's explore the diverse offerings of this tropical treasure.

Nutrient-Rich Coconut Meat: The white, fleshy part of the coconut, known as coconut meat, is rich in nutrients. A one-cup serving of shredded coconut meat (about 93 grams) provides approximately:

- Calories: 283

- Protein: 3 grams

- Fiber: 7 grams

- Healthy Fats: 27 grams (including medium-chain triglycerides, MCTs)

- Manganese: 67% of the Recommended Daily Allowance (RDA)

- Copper: 22% of the RDA

- Iron: 11% of the RDA

Hydrating Coconut Water: Found inside young, green coconuts, coconut water is a natural hydrator packed with electrolytes. It's low in calories, fat-free, and provides potassium, magnesium, and calcium.

Heart-Healthy MCTs: Coconut oil is a rich source of medium-chain triglycerides (MCTs), which are fats that the body can quickly metabolize for energy. MCTs have been associated with various health benefits, including improved cognitive function and weight management.

Antioxidant Properties: Coconut contains antioxidants, such as phenolic compounds, which help combat oxidative stress and inflammation in the body. These properties contribute to overall health and may have anti-aging effects.

Hair and Skin Nourishment: Coconut oil is a popular natural remedy for hair and skin care. Its moisturizing properties make it a common ingredient in hair conditioners, lotions, and skincare products.

Culinary Versatility: Coconut adds a distinct flavor and texture to a wide range of dishes. Some popular uses include:

- Coconut Milk: Extracted from grated coconut meat, it is a common ingredient in curries, soups, and desserts.

- Coconut Oil: Used for cooking, baking, and frying. It has a high smoke point, making it suitable for various culinary applications.

- Coconut Flour: Ground from dried coconut meat, it's a gluten-free alternative in baking.

- Desiccated Coconut: Finely shredded coconut used in baking and confectionery.

- Coconut Water: Enjoyed as a refreshing beverage on its own or used as a base for smoothies and cocktails.

Immune Support: The lauric acid found in coconut has antimicrobial and antiviral properties, which may contribute to immune system support. It is converted into monolaurin in the body, known for its potential antiviral effects.

Sustainable Crop: Coconut palms are highly resilient and can thrive in a variety of tropical environments. They are known for their sustainable nature, as almost every part of the coconut palm can be utilized.

Cultural Significance: Coconut holds cultural significance in many tropical regions, where it plays a central role in culinary traditions, religious ceremonies, and daily life.

Considerations: While coconut is nutrient-rich, it is also calorie-dense, so moderation is key, especially for individuals watching their calorie intake. Additionally, coconut products should be chosen wisely, considering factors like processing methods and added ingredients.

Conclusion:

Coconut, with its versatile offerings and nutritional richness, is a testament to the bounty that tropical regions provide. From its hydrating water to its nourishing meat and oil, coconut has ingrained itself in culinary traditions and daily rituals around the world. As we indulge in its flavors and reap the benefits it offers, coconut stands tall as a symbol of both exotic indulgence and wholesome nourishment.

Cucumber

Cucumber, with its high water content and refreshing crunch, is a widely enjoyed vegetable that adds a cooling element to various dishes. Belonging to the gourd family, cucumbers are not only hydrating but also a source of essential nutrients. Let's explore the many facets of this humble yet versatile vegetable.

Hydration Hero: Cucumbers are composed of about 95% water, making them an excellent hydrating option, especially on hot days. Incorporating cucumbers into your diet is a tasty way to stay refreshed.

Nutrient Profile: While low in calories, cucumbers offer a variety of essential nutrients. A one-cup serving of sliced cucumbers (about 119 grams) provides approximately:

- Calories: 16

- Vitamin K: 14% of the Recommended Daily Allowance (RDA)

- Vitamin C: 4% of the RDA

- Potassium: 4% of the RDA

- Dietary Fiber: 1 gram

Antioxidant Content: Cucumbers contain antioxidants, including beta-carotene and flavonoids, which help combat oxidative stress and inflammation. These compounds contribute to overall health and may play a role in disease prevention.

Skin and Hair Benefits: Cucumbers are a common ingredient in skincare routines. The silica content in cucumbers is believed to contribute to skin health, promoting hydration and elasticity. Cucumber slices are also used to reduce puffiness around the eyes.

Weight Management: Due to their high water and low-calorie content, cucumbers are a satisfying and crunchy snack for those watching their weight. They add bulk to meals without adding excess calories.

Digestive Aid: The fiber in cucumbers supports digestive health by promoting regular bowel movements and preventing constipation. Including cucumbers in your diet can contribute to a healthy gut.

Versatile Culinary Uses: Cucumbers lend themselves to a variety of culinary applications, offering a crisp texture and mild flavor. Some popular ways to enjoy cucumbers include:

- Fresh in Salads: Sliced or diced cucumbers add a refreshing element to salads.

- Pickles: Cucumbers can be preserved through pickling, resulting in a tangy and crunchy snack.

- Cucumber Water: Infusing water with cucumber slices adds a subtle flavor and encourages hydration.

- Tzatziki Sauce: A popular Mediterranean sauce made with yogurt, garlic, and finely chopped cucumbers.

- Cucumber Rolls: Sliced cucumbers can be filled and rolled with various ingredients for a creative and healthy snack.

Low in Saturated Fat and Cholesterol: Cucumbers are naturally low in saturated fat and cholesterol, making them a heart-healthy option as part of a balanced diet.

Culinary Complement: Cucumbers act as a neutral base, complementing a wide range of flavors. Their versatility allows them to be paired with both savory and sweet ingredients.

Easy to Grow: Cucumbers are relatively easy to grow, making them a popular choice for home gardens. Their vines produce an abundance of cucumbers during the growing season.

Conclusion:

Cucumber, with its high water content and nutrient profile, embodies simplicity and wellness. Whether sliced into a refreshing salad or enjoyed as a hydrating snack, cucumbers offer a delightful combination of crispness and mild flavor. As a versatile vegetable that contributes to both culinary enjoyment and overall health, cucumbers remind us that sometimes, the simplest pleasures are the most rewarding.

Eggplant

Eggplant, also known as aubergine, is a unique and versatile vegetable that has found its way into cuisines around the world. With its distinctive glossy skin and mild flavor, eggplant serves as a blank canvas for a variety of culinary creations. Beyond its culinary appeal, eggplant boasts a range of nutrients that contribute to a well-rounded and healthful diet.

Nutrient-Rich Profile: Eggplant is low in calories but rich in essential nutrients. A one-cup serving of cooked eggplant (about 82 grams) provides approximately:

- Calories: 20

- Fiber: 2.5 grams

- Vitamin C: 2% of the Recommended Daily Allowance (RDA)

- Vitamin K: 3% of the RDA

- Folate (Vitamin B9): 2% of the RDA

- Potassium: 3% of the RDA

- Manganese: 5% of the RDA

Rich in Antioxidants: Eggplant contains antioxidants, including nasunin, which may help protect cells from damage caused by free radicals. Antioxidants contribute to overall health and may have anti-inflammatory effects.

Dietary Fiber for Digestive Health: The fiber content in eggplant supports digestive health by promoting regular bowel movements and preventing constipation. Fiber also helps maintain a healthy gut microbiome.

Heart-Healthy Potassium: Eggplant is a good source of potassium, a mineral that plays a crucial role in heart health. Potassium helps regulate blood pressure and supports proper heart function.

Weight Management: With its low calorie and high fiber content, eggplant is a filling and satisfying vegetable that can be included in weight management and calorie-conscious diets.

Versatile Culinary Uses: Eggplant's neutral flavor and unique texture make it a versatile ingredient in various dishes. Some popular ways to enjoy eggplant include:

- Grilled or Roasted: Enhances its natural sweetness and imparts a smoky flavor.

- Stuffed: Filled with a mixture of grains, vegetables, and seasonings.

- Baked or Fried: Used in dishes like eggplant parmesan or moussaka.

- Pureed: Blended into dips or spreads, such as baba ganoush.

- Sautéed: Added to stir-fries or pasta dishes.

Low in Saturated Fat and Cholesterol: Eggplant is naturally low in saturated fat and cholesterol, making it a heart-healthy choice as part of a balanced diet.

Culinary Substitutes: Eggplant can be a creative substitute in recipes, such as using eggplant slices as a low-carb alternative to lasagna noodles or as a meat substitute in vegetarian dishes.

Variety of Types: There are various types of eggplant, each with its unique size, shape, and color. Common varieties include the large and dark purple globe eggplant, slender Japanese eggplant, and the small and round Thai eggplant.

Global Culinary Presence: Eggplant is a staple in many cuisines, from Mediterranean dishes like ratatouille to Middle Eastern specialties like baba ganoush and Indian curries. Its adaptability makes it a favorite in both vegetarian and non-vegetarian recipes.

Conclusion:

Eggplant, with its mild flavor and nutrient richness, shines as a versatile and nutritious addition to our culinary repertoire. As we explore the many ways to prepare and enjoy eggplant, we not only savor its unique taste and texture but also benefit from the valuable nutrients it brings to the table. Whether grilled, roasted, or pureed, eggplant stands as a testament to the delightful fusion of flavor and health in the world of vegetables.

Figs

Figs, with their luscious sweetness and unique texture, are ancient fruits celebrated for both their culinary and health benefits. These teardrop-shaped delights are not only delicious when enjoyed fresh or dried but also offer a wealth of essential nutrients. Let's explore the rich tapestry of flavors and goodness that figs bring to the table.

Nutrient-Packed Sweetness: Figs are dense with essential nutrients, making them a satisfying and wholesome snack. A one-cup serving of fresh figs (about 151 grams) provides approximately:

- Calories: 107

- Dietary Fiber: 7.4 grams

- Vitamin K: 33% of the Recommended Daily Allowance (RDA)

- Vitamin B6: 6% of the RDA

- Copper: 10% of the RDA

- Manganese: 9% of the RDA

- Potassium: 9% of the RDA

Natural Sugar and Energy: Figs are a natural source of sweetness, primarily from natural sugars like glucose, fructose, and sucrose. This natural sweetness, combined with fiber, provides a sustained release of energy.

Rich in Dietary Fiber: Figs are an excellent source of dietary fiber, promoting digestive health and aiding in weight management. Fiber adds bulk to the stool, prevents constipation, and supports a healthy gut microbiome.

Antioxidant Properties: Figs contain antioxidants, including polyphenols and flavonoids, which help neutralize free radicals in the body. These antioxidants contribute to overall health and may have anti-inflammatory effects.

Heart Health: The potassium content in figs supports heart health by helping regulate blood pressure. Additionally, the dietary fiber in figs contributes to lower cholesterol levels, reducing the risk of cardiovascular diseases.

Iron for Blood Health: Figs are a good source of iron, a vital mineral for the formation of red blood cells and oxygen transport in the body. Including figs in the diet can contribute to maintaining optimal blood health.

Calcium for Bone Health: Figs contain calcium, essential for bone health and preventing conditions like osteoporosis. Calcium is crucial for maintaining strong and healthy bones.

Versatile Culinary Uses: Figs are incredibly versatile in the kitchen, adding a touch of sweetness to both sweet and savory dishes. Some popular ways to enjoy figs include:

- Fresh: Enjoyed on their own or added to salads for a burst of natural sweetness.

- Dried: A classic snack or used in baking, desserts, and trail mixes.

- Fig Jam or Preserves: Spread on toast or paired with cheese for a delightful appetizer.

- Grilled or Roasted: Enhances their natural sweetness and pairs well with savory dishes.

- In Yogurt or Smoothies: Adds a natural sweetener and texture to breakfast or snacks.

Seasonal and Global Appeal: Figs have a seasonality that varies by region, making them a sought-after delicacy during their peak freshness. They are enjoyed in various cuisines globally, from Mediterranean to Middle Eastern and beyond.

Ancient Symbolism: Figs have historical and symbolic significance in many cultures. They are often associated with abundance, fertility, and sweetness, playing a role in various traditions and rituals.

Conclusion:

Figs, with their sumptuous sweetness and nutritional richness, offer a delightful fusion of taste and health benefits. As we relish the unique texture and flavor of figs, we also embrace the wealth of nutrients they provide. Whether enjoyed fresh, dried, or incorporated into culinary creations, figs stand as a testament to the inherent goodness and indulgence found in nature's bountiful offerings.

Garlic

Garlic, with its unmistakable aroma and bold flavor, has been a culinary and medicinal staple for centuries. Belonging to the Allium family, along with onions and leeks, garlic is celebrated for its ability to transform dishes and contribute to a wide array of health benefits. Let's explore the versatile nature of this pungent bulb.

Nutrient-Rich Composition: Garlic is a nutrient-dense bulb, providing essential vitamins and minerals. A one-clove serving (about 3 grams) offers approximately:

  - Calories: 4

  - Vitamin C: 2% of the Recommended Daily Allowance (RDA)

  - Manganese: 2% of the RDA

  - B6 (Pyridoxine): 2% of the RDA

Allicin and Sulphur Compounds: The characteristic pungency of garlic is attributed to allicin, a sulfur-containing compound formed when garlic is crushed or chopped. Allicin is known for its potential health benefits, including anti-bacterial and anti-inflammatory properties.

Immune System Support: Garlic has been traditionally valued for its immune-boosting properties. Its allicin content, along with other compounds, may contribute to enhanced immune function, helping the body defend against infections.

Heart Health: Garlic is associated with cardiovascular benefits. It may help lower blood pressure, reduce cholesterol levels, and improve overall heart health. Allicin's antioxidant properties contribute to the prevention of oxidative stress on the cardiovascular system.

Anti-Inflammatory Effects: Garlic contains compounds that exhibit anti-inflammatory effects, potentially aiding in the management of inflammatory conditions and reducing the risk of chronic diseases.

Antimicrobial and Antibacterial Properties: Garlic has been used traditionally for its antimicrobial properties. Allicin and other sulfur compounds in garlic may have antibacterial and antiviral effects, making it a natural remedy for various ailments.

Digestive Aid: Garlic may support digestive health by promoting the growth of beneficial gut bacteria. It also has mild laxative properties that can aid in regular bowel movements.

Culinary Versatility: Garlic's culinary applications are vast, enhancing the flavor of a wide range of dishes. Some popular uses include:

  - Sautéed or Roasted: Adds depth and aroma to savory dishes.

  - Raw: Finely minced in salads, dressings, or sauces for a potent kick.

  - Pickled or Fermented: As seen in pickled garlic or garlic-infused condiments.

  - In Soups and Stews: A staple ingredient for rich and flavorful broths.

Historical Significance: Garlic has a rich history, dating back to ancient civilizations. It was used for culinary and medicinal purposes in cultures such as Ancient Egypt, Greece, and Rome.

Garlic was even employed during World War I and World War II as an antiseptic to prevent wound infections.

Superstitions and Folklore: Throughout history, garlic has been surrounded by superstitions and folklore. It was believed to ward off evil spirits, vampires, and the plague. Despite its pungent odor, garlic was considered a protective charm in many cultures.

Conclusion:

Garlic, with its potent aroma and myriad health benefits, stands as a testament to the dual role of many culinary herbs and spices. As a staple in kitchens worldwide, garlic not only elevates the taste of dishes but also contributes to overall well-being. Whether used as a flavor enhancer or a natural remedy, garlic continues to weave its aromatic and beneficial magic into the fabric of culinary traditions and health practices.

Ginger

Ginger, with its warm and zesty flavor, is a versatile rhizome that has played a central role in culinary and medicinal traditions for centuries. Known for its aromatic profile and potential health benefits, ginger adds a distinctive kick to dishes and has been valued for its therapeutic properties. Let's delve into the multifaceted world of this remarkable spice.

Nutrient-Rich Composition: Ginger is rich in bioactive compounds and essential nutrients. A one-ounce (28 grams) serving provides approximately:

- Calories: 23

- Dietary Fiber: 2 grams

- Carbohydrates: 5 grams

- Sugars: 0.1 grams

- Vitamin C: 1% of the Recommended Daily Allowance (RDA)

- Vitamin B6: 1% of the RDA

- Iron: 1% of the RDA

- Potassium: 1% of the RDA

Gingerol and Bioactive Compounds: The bioactive compound responsible for ginger's distinct flavor and potential health benefits is gingerol. Gingerol has antioxidant and anti-inflammatory properties, contributing to its medicinal value.

Digestive Comfort: Ginger has long been revered for its digestive benefits. It can help alleviate nausea, including morning sickness during pregnancy and nausea induced by chemotherapy. Gingerol is thought to relax the gastrointestinal muscles and reduce irritation.

Anti-Inflammatory Effects: The anti-inflammatory properties of ginger can be beneficial for managing various inflammatory conditions, such as osteoarthritis and rheumatoid arthritis. It may help alleviate joint pain and improve mobility.

Immune-Boosting Qualities: Ginger has immune-boosting potential due to its antioxidant content. Regular consumption may contribute to overall immune system support and resilience against infections.

Motion Sickness and Morning Sickness Relief: Ginger has been studied for its effectiveness in reducing motion sickness and morning sickness. It can be consumed in various forms, including ginger tea or ginger candies, to help mitigate these discomforts.

Culinary Versatility: Ginger's versatility in the kitchen is showcased in a variety of culinary applications. Some popular uses include:

- Freshly Grated: Adds a zesty kick to stir-fries, soups, and marinades.

- Ground Ginger: Used in baking, spice blends, and desserts.

- Ginger Tea: A soothing and invigorating beverage.

- Pickled Ginger: Often served with sushi to cleanse the palate.

- Ginger Syrup: A sweet and spicy addition to beverages and cocktails.

Asian Culinary Staple: Ginger is a foundational ingredient in many Asian cuisines, where its aromatic and warming qualities are highly valued. It is a key component in dishes ranging from curries to stir-fries.

Traditional Medicine: In traditional medicine, ginger has been used to address various ailments, including colds, headaches, and digestive issues. Its historical use in herbal remedies has persisted across cultures.

Culinary and Medicinal Harmony: The dual nature of ginger, seamlessly transitioning between culinary delight and medicinal remedy, highlights its unique place in both the kitchen and the apothecary. Its ability to enhance the flavor of dishes while offering potential health benefits makes it a prized addition to a well-rounded lifestyle.

Conclusion:

Ginger, with its lively flavor and therapeutic potential, stands as a testament to the harmonious relationship between culinary herbs and health-promoting spices. Whether embraced for its culinary versatility or valued for its potential medicinal properties, ginger continues to captivate and enrich our sensory and well-being experiences. As a spice that transcends cultural boundaries, ginger's timeless appeal persists, inviting us to savor its zest and embrace its potential for vitality and balance.

Grapes

Grapes, with their sweet and juicy allure, have been a beloved fruit for millennia. Whether enjoyed fresh, dried into raisins, or transformed into wine, grapes offer a delightful burst of flavor along with an array of health benefits. Let's explore the wonders of these bite-sized jewels from nature.

Nutrient-Rich Goodness: Grapes are not only delicious but also packed with essential nutrients. A one-cup serving of grapes (about 151 grams) provides approximately:

- Calories: 104

- Carbohydrates: 27 grams

- Dietary Fiber: 1.4 grams

- Vitamin K: 22% of the Recommended Daily Allowance (RDA)

- Vitamin C: 27% of the RDA

- Copper: 10% of the RDA

- Potassium: 8% of the RDA

Antioxidant Powerhouse: Grapes are rich in antioxidants, including resveratrol, quercetin, and anthocyanins. These compounds help neutralize free radicals, protect cells from damage, and contribute to overall health.

Heart Health: Resveratrol, found in grape skins, has been associated with cardiovascular benefits. It may help lower blood pressure, reduce inflammation, and improve cholesterol levels, contributing to heart health.

Immune Support: The vitamin C content in grapes supports the immune system by promoting the production of white blood cells and enhancing the body's ability to fight infections.

Hydration and Dietary Fiber: With a high water content and dietary fiber, grapes contribute to hydration and digestive health. Fiber aids in regular bowel movements and helps maintain a healthy gut.

Grapes and Wine: Grapes are a key ingredient in winemaking, contributing to the vast array of wines available worldwide. Red wine, in particular, is known for its potential heart-protective effects attributed to compounds like resveratrol.

Variety of Types: Grapes come in various colors and types, each offering a unique flavor profile. Common varieties include red grapes (e.g., Cabernet Sauvignon), green grapes (e.g., Thompson Seedless), and black grapes (e.g., Concord).

Culinary Versatility: Grapes are a versatile ingredient in both sweet and savory dishes. Some popular ways to enjoy grapes include:

- Fresh: Eaten as a snack or added to fruit salads.

- Dried: Raisins, sultanas, and currants are popular dried grape varieties used in baking, trail mixes, and desserts.

- Juice and Smoothies: Blended into refreshing beverages.

- Wine: Enjoyed in its various forms, from red and white to sparkling and dessert wines.

- Jellies and Jams: Used to make spreads and condiments.

Seasonal Delight: Grapes are often associated with late summer and early fall, making them a seasonal delight. The harvest season is celebrated in many cultures with festivals and events.

Symbolism and Traditions: Grapes hold symbolic significance in various cultures and traditions. They are often associated with abundance, prosperity, and celebration. In many cultures, grapes are a part of New Year's Eve traditions, symbolizing good luck and a fruitful year ahead.

Conclusion:

Grapes, with their succulent sweetness and nutrient richness, stand as a testament to the simple joys and healthful offerings found in nature. As we pop these juicy jewels into our mouths or savor a fine glass of wine, we not only indulge in a delightful culinary experience but also partake in the age-old celebration of a fruit that has woven itself into the fabric of human history and culture.

Green Beans

Green beans, also known as snap beans or string beans, are crisp, vibrant pods that belong to the legume family. Loved for their tender texture and mild flavor, green beans are not only a versatile ingredient in various culinary dishes but also offer an array of essential nutrients. Let's explore the delightful world of these green gems.

Nutrient-Rich Composition: Green beans are a low-calorie, nutrient-dense vegetable, providing a variety of essential vitamins and minerals. A one-cup serving of cooked green beans (about 125 grams) offers approximately:

- Calories: 31

- Protein: 1.8 grams

- Dietary Fiber: 3.4 grams

- Vitamin C: 14% of the Recommended Daily Allowance (RDA)

- Vitamin K: 19% of the RDA

- Folate (Vitamin B9): 10% of the RDA

- Manganese: 9% of the RDA

Antioxidant Power: Green beans contain various antioxidants, such as beta-carotene and flavonoids, which help neutralize free radicals in the body. Antioxidants contribute to overall health and may have anti-inflammatory effects.

Heart Health: The fiber, potassium, and folate content in green beans support heart health. Fiber helps manage cholesterol levels, potassium regulates blood pressure, and folate contributes to the prevention of homocysteine buildup in the blood vessels.

Blood Sugar Regulation: The fiber in green beans aids in slowing down the absorption of sugars, contributing to better blood sugar regulation. This makes green beans a suitable choice for individuals managing diabetes.

Digestive Health: Green beans are a good source of dietary fiber, which promotes healthy digestion. Fiber adds bulk to stool, prevents constipation, and supports a balanced gut microbiome.

Versatile Culinary Uses: Green beans lend themselves to a variety of culinary applications, offering a satisfying crunch and mild flavor. Some popular ways to enjoy green beans include:

- Steamed or Blanched: Retains their vibrant color and crisp texture.

- Sautéed or Stir-Fried: Adds depth of flavor with various seasonings and spices.

- Roasted: Enhances their natural sweetness and imparts a smoky flavor.

- In Salads: A refreshing addition to green salads or grain bowls.

- As a Side Dish: Boiled and served as a simple yet nutritious side.

Varieties of Green Beans: There are different varieties of green beans, including traditional string beans, French haricots verts, and the flatter Italian Romano beans. Each variety offers a slightly different taste and texture.

Easy to Grow: Green beans are a popular choice for home gardens. They are relatively easy to grow and thrive in a variety of climates. Both bush and pole varieties are available.

Seasonal Availability: Green beans are often associated with the summer season when they are harvested at their peak freshness. However, they are available in supermarkets year-round.

Nutrient Preservation: To preserve the maximum nutritional value, it's recommended to cook green beans using methods that retain their vibrant color and crispness, such as steaming or blanching.

Conclusion:

Green beans, with their vibrant color and nutrient-packed profile, are a delightful addition to a well-balanced diet. As a versatile vegetable, they contribute not only to culinary creativity but also to the promotion of overall health. Whether enjoyed fresh, sautéed, or tossed in a salad, green beans stand as a testament to the simple yet powerful impact that wholesome, plant-based foods can have on our well-being.

Kale

Kale, a leafy green vegetable, has earned its reputation as a nutritional powerhouse and a versatile culinary ingredient. With its robust flavor and abundance of essential nutrients, kale has become a favorite among health-conscious individuals. Let's explore the many facets of kale that make it a standout in the world of leafy greens.

Nutrient-Rich Superfood: Kale is packed with essential nutrients, making it one of the most nutrient-dense foods available. A one-cup serving of raw kale (about 67 grams) provides approximately:

- Calories: 33

- Protein: 2.2 grams

- Dietary Fiber: 1.3 grams

- Vitamin A: 206% of the Recommended Daily Allowance (RDA)

- Vitamin C: 134% of the RDA

- Vitamin K: 684% of the RDA

- Calcium: 9% of the RDA

- Iron: 6% of the RDA

High in Antioxidants: Kale is rich in antioxidants, including beta-carotene, flavonoids, and polyphenols. These compounds help neutralize free radicals in the body, contributing to overall health and potentially reducing the risk of chronic diseases.

Vitamin K for Bone Health: The exceptionally high vitamin K content in kale is essential for bone health. Vitamin K plays a crucial role in calcium absorption and bone mineralization, contributing to bone strength.

Abundant Vitamin C: Kale is an excellent source of vitamin C, an antioxidant that supports the immune system, promotes skin health, and aids in collagen production.

Iron for Energy: While the iron content in plant-based foods like kale is non-heme iron (less easily absorbed than heme iron from animal sources), the presence of vitamin C in kale enhances iron absorption, contributing to energy production and preventing iron deficiency.

Healthy Fats and Omega-3s: Kale contains small amounts of healthy fats, including omega-3 fatty acids. These fats are beneficial for heart health, inflammation reduction, and brain function.

Digestive Support: The fiber content in kale promotes healthy digestion, supports regular bowel movements, and contributes to gut health. Fiber also helps in maintaining a feeling of fullness, making kale a valuable addition to weight management diets.

Versatile Culinary Uses: Kale's versatility makes it a popular ingredient in various dishes. Some popular ways to enjoy kale include:

- Raw in Salads: Massaging kale leaves with a dressing can soften them and make for a flavorful salad.

- Sauteed or Stir-Fried: Adds a robust flavor to savory dishes.

- Blended in Smoothies: Incorporates the nutritional benefits of kale into a refreshing beverage.

- Baked into Chips: Kale chips make for a crunchy and nutritious snack.

Different Varieties: There are different varieties of kale, including curly kale, lacinato (or dinosaur) kale, and red or Russian kale. Each variety has its unique taste and texture.

Cold-Weather Resilience: Kale is known for its hardiness and ability to thrive in colder climates. In fact, its flavor can even improve after exposure to frost, making it a reliable source of greens during the winter months.

Conclusion:

Kale, with its exceptional nutrient profile and culinary versatility, stands as a symbol of the nutritional bounty that nature provides. Whether enjoyed in salads, sautéed dishes, or blended into smoothies, kale offers a robust and healthful addition to our diets. As a leafy green that reigns supreme in both flavor and nutrition, kale continues to hold its place as a cornerstone in the world of wholesome and plant-based eating.

Kiwi

Kiwi, also known as the Chinese gooseberry, is a small, vibrant fruit that packs a punch when it comes to flavor and nutrition. With its unique combination of sweet and tangy taste, along with an impressive array of essential nutrients, kiwi has become a popular addition to fruit bowls, salads, and snacks around the world. Let's explore the delightful qualities that make kiwi a standout in the world of fruits.

Vitamin C Powerhouse: Kiwi is renowned for its exceptionally high vitamin C content. A one-cup serving of sliced kiwi (about 177 grams) provides approximately:

- Calories: 108

- Vitamin C: 273% of the Recommended Daily Allowance (RDA)

- Vitamin K: 31% of the RDA

- Dietary Fiber: 5.4 grams

- Folate (Vitamin B9): 10% of the RDA

- Potassium: 14% of the RDA

Antioxidant Richness: Kiwi is packed with antioxidants, including vitamin C, vitamin E, and polyphenols. These antioxidants help combat oxidative stress, protect cells from damage, and contribute to overall health.

Fiber for Digestive Health: The dietary fiber in kiwi supports digestive health by promoting regular bowel movements, preventing constipation, and contributing to a healthy gut microbiome.

Heart-Healthy Potassium: Kiwi contains potassium, a mineral that plays a key role in maintaining heart health by regulating blood pressure and supporting proper cardiovascular function.

Immune System Support: The combination of vitamin C, vitamin K, and other antioxidants in kiwi supports the immune system, helping the body defend against infections and illnesses.

Skin and Hair Benefits: The vitamin C content in kiwi is essential for collagen synthesis, promoting healthy skin and hair. Collagen is a structural protein that contributes to skin elasticity and strength.

Low in Calories, High in Nutrients: Kiwi is a nutrient-dense fruit, meaning it provides a significant amount of vitamins and minerals relative to its calorie content. This makes it a healthy choice for those looking to maximize nutrient intake.

Unique Flavor and Texture: Kiwi offers a distinctive combination of sweetness and tartness, coupled with a unique texture that includes tiny, edible black seeds. The contrast of flavors and textures makes kiwi a delightful addition to fruit salads and desserts.

Culinary Versatility: Kiwi can be enjoyed in various ways, including:

- Fresh and Raw: Peeled and sliced for a refreshing snack or added to fruit salads.

- Blended in Smoothies: Enhances the flavor and nutritional content of smoothie recipes.

- As a Garnish: Sliced or diced to decorate desserts, yogurt, or breakfast bowls.

Seasonal and Global Availability: While kiwi has its peak season, it is available in grocery stores year-round due to its cultivation in different regions around the world. This availability ensures a consistent supply of this nutritious fruit.

Conclusion:

Kiwi, with its bold flavor and nutritional richness, stands as a vibrant jewel in the world of fruits. As a versatile and healthful addition to a balanced diet, kiwi invites us to savor its unique taste while reaping the benefits of its impressive nutrient profile. Whether enjoyed on its own or incorporated into various culinary creations, kiwi continues to captivate taste buds and contribute to the colorful palette of wholesome eating.

Leeks

Leeks, with their mild onion flavor and distinctive cylindrical shape, are versatile vegetables that add depth and complexity to a variety of dishes. Belonging to the Allium family, which also includes onions and garlic, leeks bring a unique taste and nutritional profile to the table. Let's explore the culinary and health attributes that make leeks a standout in the world of vegetables.

Nutrient-Rich Composition: Leeks are a low-calorie vegetable that offers a range of essential nutrients. A one-cup serving of chopped leeks (about 89 grams) provides approximately:

- Calories: 54

- Dietary Fiber: 1.6 grams

- Vitamin K: 29% of the Recommended Daily Allowance (RDA)

- Vitamin C: 14% of the RDA

- Folate (Vitamin B9): 10% of the RDA

- Manganese: 9% of the RDA

Mild Onion Flavor: Leeks have a milder and sweeter taste compared to onions, making them a versatile ingredient in various culinary creations. They add a subtle onion flavor without overpowering the dish.

Digestive Health: The fiber content in leeks supports digestive health by promoting regular bowel movements and preventing constipation. Fiber also contributes to a healthy gut microbiome.

Antioxidant Properties: Leeks contain antioxidants, including polyphenols and flavonoids, which help neutralize free radicals in the body. Antioxidants contribute to overall health and may have anti-inflammatory effects.

Vitamin K for Bone Health: The significant vitamin K content in leeks is crucial for bone health. Vitamin K plays a key role in proper blood clotting and bone mineralization.

Vitamin C for Immune Support: Leeks provide a notable amount of vitamin C, supporting the immune system, promoting skin health, and aiding in collagen production.

Culinary Versatility: Leeks can be used in various culinary applications, adding flavor and texture to dishes. Some popular ways to enjoy leeks include:

  - Sautéed or Stir-Fried: Enhances the mild onion flavor and creates a savory base for many dishes.

  - In Soups and Stews: Adds depth to broths and complements other vegetables and proteins.

  - Grilled or Roasted: Develops a caramelized sweetness and a slightly crispy texture.

  - In Casseroles or Quiches: Adds a unique taste to baked dishes.

Leek Greens and Whites: Leeks consist of both white and green parts. The white part is typically used in cooking, while the green part can be used for making stock or discarded. However, both parts are edible and nutritious.

Growing Leeks: Leeks are often grown in cooler climates and are known for their resilience in colder temperatures. They are typically planted as seedlings and can be harvested once they reach the desired size.

Mediterranean and European Cuisine: Leeks have a significant presence in Mediterranean and European cuisines, where they are featured in classic dishes such as vichyssoise (a chilled leek and potato soup) and quiche.

Conclusion:

Leeks, with their mild and sweet onion flavor, contribute to a wide range of dishes, adding depth and nutritional value. As a nutrient-rich vegetable, leeks offer a delicious way to enhance the taste and healthfulness of meals. Whether sautéed, roasted, or simmered in soups, leeks continue to hold their place as a culinary gem in the world of vegetables, inviting us to savor their distinctive taste and reap the benefits of their nutrient-packed goodness.

Lemons

Lemons, with their bright yellow hue and tangy flavor, are a versatile citrus fruit that brings zest and freshness to a variety of culinary delights. Beyond their culinary uses, lemons are known for their health-promoting properties, making them a popular addition to both sweet and savory dishes. Let's explore the vibrant world of lemons, where their taste and benefits converge.

Vitamin C Powerhouse: Lemons are renowned for their high vitamin C content, a potent antioxidant that supports the immune system, promotes skin health, and aids in collagen production. A one-cup serving of lemon juice (about 244 grams) provides approximately:

- Calories: 61

- Vitamin C: 187% of the Recommended Daily Allowance (RDA)

- Folate (Vitamin B9): 3% of the RDA

- Potassium: 3% of the RDA

Immune System Support: The abundance of vitamin C in lemons contributes to immune system health, helping the body defend against infections and illnesses. Regular consumption of lemon-infused beverages or dishes provides a natural boost to the immune system.

Antioxidant Properties: Lemons contain various antioxidants, including flavonoids, which help neutralize free radicals in the body. Antioxidants play a crucial role in reducing oxidative stress and promoting overall health.

Digestive Aid: Lemon water is a popular choice for many as a morning beverage. The acidity of lemons, combined with warm water, may help stimulate digestion and promote healthy bowel movements.

Alkalizing Effect: Despite being acidic in nature, lemons have an alkalizing effect on the body. This can help balance the body's pH levels and create an environment less conducive to inflammation.

Culinary Versatility: Lemons are incredibly versatile in the kitchen, enhancing both sweet and savory dishes. Some popular ways to enjoy lemons include:

- Lemonade: A classic and refreshing beverage, especially in warmer months.

- Salad Dressings: Squeezed over salads for a burst of citrusy flavor.

- Marinades: Used to tenderize and flavor meats, fish, and vegetables.

- Desserts: Lemon is a common flavor in cakes, pies, tarts, and sorbets.

- Tea: A slice of lemon can be added to hot or cold tea for extra flavor.

Essential Oil and Aromatherapy: Lemon essential oil, extracted from the peel, is used in aromatherapy for its invigorating and uplifting scent. It's also a popular addition to natural cleaning products.

Skincare Benefits: The vitamin C and antioxidants in lemons contribute to skin health. Lemon juice is sometimes used topically for its astringent and brightening properties. However, caution is advised due to its acidity, which may irritate sensitive skin.

Weight Management: The fiber content in lemons, particularly in the pulp, may contribute to a feeling of fullness, making them a potentially beneficial addition to weight management diets.

Symbolic Significance: Lemons are often associated with cleanliness and freshness. They symbolize purity and are commonly used in cleaning products for their pleasant scent and antibacterial properties.

Conclusion:

Lemons, with their invigorating flavor and healthful properties, stand as a testament to the remarkable benefits that nature's citrus bounty brings to our lives. From culinary creations to wellness routines, lemons continue to play a vibrant and refreshing role, inspiring us to savor their zesty essence and embrace the multitude of ways they contribute to our taste buds and well-being.

Lettuce

Lettuce, with its tender leaves and refreshing crunch, is a staple in the world of leafy greens. This humble yet versatile vegetable serves as the base for countless salads, wraps, and sandwiches, contributing not only to culinary creations but also to a nutrient-packed diet. Let's explore the qualities that make lettuce a favorite in the realm of fresh and vibrant greens.

Variety of Types: Lettuce comes in various types, each offering a unique texture and flavor. Common varieties include:

- Iceberg Lettuce: Known for its crisp and mild taste, with tightly packed leaves.

- Romaine Lettuce: Characterized by long, sturdy leaves and a slightly bitter taste.

- Butterhead (e.g., Bibb and Boston): Features loose, tender leaves with a buttery texture.

- Leaf Lettuce (e.g., Red Leaf and Green Leaf): Offers loose, frilly leaves with a mild flavor.

- Arugula: A peppery, dark green leafy green often included in salad mixes.

Low in Calories, High in Nutrients: Lettuce is low in calories, making it an excellent choice for those looking to maintain or lose weight. It's also a good source of essential nutrients, including:

- Vitamin K: Crucial for blood clotting and bone health.

- Vitamin A: Important for vision, skin health, and immune function.

- Folate (Vitamin B9): Essential for DNA synthesis and cell growth.

Hydration and Fiber: With a high water content, lettuce contributes to hydration. Additionally, the fiber in lettuce supports digestive health by adding bulk to stool and promoting regular bowel movements.

Antioxidant Properties: While not as rich in antioxidants as some other vegetables, lettuce does contain compounds that contribute to its overall health benefits. Antioxidants help neutralize free radicals and protect cells from damage.

Culinary Versatility: Lettuce serves as a versatile ingredient in a variety of dishes, beyond traditional salads. Some common uses include:

- Wraps and Tacos: Large lettuce leaves can be used as a substitute for tortillas.

- Burgers and Sandwiches: Adds a crisp and refreshing layer to sandwiches.

- Soups and Stir-Fries: Certain types of lettuce can be added to hot dishes for a mild flavor and texture.

Seasonal Availability: Lettuce is generally available year-round, with different varieties flourishing in various seasons. Its widespread cultivation ensures a consistent supply in grocery stores.

Farm-to-Table Freshness: Lettuce is often enjoyed in its freshest state, as it can be consumed raw. Its farm-to-table journey allows for optimal taste and nutritional value.

Hydroponic and Indoor Cultivation: Advances in agriculture have enabled the cultivation of lettuce through hydroponics and indoor farming, providing a sustainable and controlled environment for year-round production.

Quick and Easy to Prepare: Lettuce requires minimal preparation, usually just washing and tearing or chopping. Its simplicity makes it an accessible choice for quick, healthy meals.

Dietary Inclusion: Lettuce is a common component of many dietary plans, including vegetarian, vegan, and low-carb diets. Its versatility and nutritional content make it a go-to option for those seeking a light and healthy foundation for meals.

Conclusion:

Lettuce, with its crisp texture and mild flavor, stands as a cornerstone in the world of leafy greens. As a nutritious and versatile vegetable, it provides a canvas for culinary creativity while contributing to a well-balanced and healthful diet. Whether served in a classic salad, wrapped around savory fillings, or added to various dishes, lettuce continues to be a refreshing and essential component of diverse cuisines worldwide.

Macadamia Nuts

Macadamia nuts, native to Australia but now enjoyed worldwide, are celebrated for their rich, buttery flavor and unique nutritional profile. These creamy delights not only make for a delicious snack but also offer a range of health benefits. Let's explore the characteristics, nutritional value, and culinary uses that make macadamia nuts a standout in the world of nuts.

Unique Flavor and Texture: Macadamia nuts are known for their distinctive taste—a buttery, smooth flavor with a hint of sweetness. Their texture is creamy and slightly crunchy, providing a delightful sensory experience.

Nutrient-Rich Composition: While macadamia nuts are calorie-dense, they are packed with beneficial nutrients. A one-ounce (28 grams) serving provides approximately:

- Calories: 204

- Total Fat: 23 grams

- Saturated Fat: 3.5 grams

- Monounsaturated Fat: 16 grams

- Protein: 2 grams

- Dietary Fiber: 2.5 grams

- Vitamin B1 (Thiamine): 12% of the Recommended Daily Allowance (RDA)

- Manganese: 58% of the RDA

Heart-Healthy Monounsaturated Fats: The majority of the fats in macadamia nuts are monounsaturated fats, particularly oleic acid. These heart-healthy fats may help reduce bad cholesterol levels and lower the risk of cardiovascular disease.

Antioxidant Properties: Macadamia nuts contain antioxidants, including tocopherols and flavonoids. These compounds help neutralize free radicals, protecting cells from oxidative stress and inflammation.

Nutrient Absorption: The monounsaturated fats in macadamia nuts may aid in the absorption of fat-soluble vitamins, such as vitamin E, which is naturally present in the nuts.

Support for Weight Management: Despite being calorie-dense, macadamia nuts may contribute to satiety due to their healthy fat and protein content. Including them in moderation as part of a balanced diet may support weight management.

Versatile Culinary Uses: Macadamia nuts are a versatile ingredient in both sweet and savory dishes. Some popular ways to enjoy them include:

- Snacking: Eaten on their own for a satisfying and nutritious snack.

- Baking: Added to cookies, cakes, and muffins for a rich and nutty flavor.

- Trail Mixes: Combined with dried fruits and other nuts for a tasty trail mix.

- Salads: Chopped or toasted macadamia nuts can enhance the texture and flavor of salads.

- Nut Butters: Blended into creamy macadamia nut butter as a delicious alternative to traditional nut butters.

Culinary Indulgence: Macadamia nuts are often considered a premium nut, valued for their unique taste and texture. They are featured in gourmet chocolates, confections, and high-end desserts.

Sustainable Farming Practices: Macadamia nuts are typically grown in subtropical regions with well-drained soil. Sustainable farming practices, including agroforestry, are employed to cultivate these trees for long-term environmental health.

Limited Geographic Production: The majority of the world's macadamia nuts come from Australia, Hawaii, and some regions in South Africa. This limited geographic production adds to the exclusivity and appeal of these nuts.

Conclusion:

Macadamia nuts, with their indulgent flavor and nutritional benefits, offer a delectable addition to a diverse range of dishes. Whether enjoyed on their own, incorporated into culinary creations, or savored in premium desserts, macadamia nuts continue to captivate taste buds and contribute to the rich tapestry of nut-based delights. As a creamy and satisfying nut variety, macadamias showcase the potential for both culinary indulgence and nutritional well-being

Mangoes

Mangoes, often hailed as the "king of fruits," are not just a seasonal delight but also a symbol of tropical indulgence. With their succulent sweetness, vibrant colors, and a rich nutritional profile, mangoes have earned their place as a beloved fruit worldwide. Let's delve into the luscious world of mangoes, exploring their flavors, nutritional benefits, and the diverse ways in which they grace our plates.

Variety of Flavors and Textures: Mangoes come in a variety of cultivars, each with its unique flavor, aroma, and texture. Some popular varieties include Alphonso, Haden, Ataulfo, and Keitt. The flavors range from intensely sweet and aromatic to mildly tart.

Nutrient-Rich Goodness: Mangoes are not only delicious but also packed with essential nutrients. A one-cup (about 225 grams) serving of diced mango provides approximately:

- Calories: 100

- Vitamin C: 60% of the Recommended Daily Allowance (RDA)

- Vitamin A: 10% of the RDA

- Fiber: 2.6 grams

- Folate (Vitamin B9): 18% of the RDA

- Vitamin E: 9% of the RDA

- Potassium: 6% of the RDA

Antioxidant Powerhouse: Mangoes are rich in antioxidants like beta-carotene, quercetin, and astragalin. These compounds help neutralize free radicals, providing potential health benefits such as reduced inflammation and protection against chronic diseases.

Immune Support: The high vitamin C content in mangoes supports the immune system by promoting the production of white blood cells and enhancing the body's ability to fight infections.

Digestive Health: Mangoes contain enzymes like amylases, which aid in breaking down carbohydrates, and fiber, which supports healthy digestion and regular bowel movements.

Heart Health: The fiber, potassium, and antioxidant content in mangoes contribute to heart health. Potassium helps regulate blood pressure, and fiber helps manage cholesterol levels.

Hydration and Refreshment: With their high water content, mangoes contribute to hydration, making them a perfect juicy treat on hot summer days.

Culinary Versatility: Mangoes are incredibly versatile in the kitchen, adding a burst of sweetness to both sweet and savory dishes. Some popular ways to enjoy mangoes include:

- Fresh and Diced: As a standalone snack or added to fruit salads.

- Smoothies: Blended into refreshing beverages for a tropical twist.

- Salsas and Chutneys: Used in savory dishes to add a sweet and tangy element.

- Desserts: Featured in ice creams, sorbets, puddings, and cakes.

- Curries and Marinades: Adds a unique flavor to savory dishes.

Cultural Significance: Mangoes hold cultural significance in many countries, symbolizing abundance, prosperity, and celebration. They are often featured in traditional ceremonies, festivals, and culinary traditions.

Seasonal Extravaganza: Mangoes are typically associated with the summer season, and their arrival is eagerly awaited as a sign of the season's vibrancy. Mango festivals and events celebrate the diversity and richness of this tropical fruit.

Conclusion:

Mangoes, with their succulent sweetness and nutrient-rich goodness, embody the essence of summer indulgence. Whether savored in their pure, juicy form or incorporated into a myriad of culinary creations, mangoes have a way of elevating the dining experience. As a symbol of tropical bounty and cultural significance, mangoes continue to capture the hearts and palates of people around the world, inviting us to savor the richness of this luscious jewel of the fruit kingdom.

Mushrooms

Mushrooms, often celebrated for their unique texture and earthy flavors, belong to the fungi kingdom and have been part of human diets for centuries. Beyond their culinary appeal, mushrooms boast a diverse range of varieties, each offering distinct tastes and nutritional benefits. Let's delve into the fascinating world of mushrooms, exploring their culinary versatility, nutritional value, and the unique role they play in various cuisines.

Culinary Versatility: Mushrooms come in various shapes, sizes, and flavors, making them incredibly versatile in the kitchen. From the meaty Portobello to the delicate enoki, mushrooms can be sautéed, roasted, grilled, stuffed, or even enjoyed raw in salads. They absorb flavors well, making them a favorite in various cuisines around the world.

Nutrient-Rich Powerhouses: Despite their low calorie content, mushrooms are packed with essential nutrients. A one-cup serving (about 70 grams) of sliced white mushrooms provides approximately:

- Calories: 15

- Protein: 2.2 grams

- Fiber: 1.1 grams

- Vitamin D: 64% of the Recommended Daily Allowance (RDA)

- Selenium: 13% of the RDA

- Riboflavin (Vitamin B2): 18% of the RDA

- Niacin (Vitamin B3): 10% of the RDA

- Copper: 12% of the RDA

Excellent Source of Vitamin D: Mushrooms exposed to sunlight or ultraviolet (UV) light naturally produce vitamin D. This makes them one of the few non-animal sources of this essential vitamin, crucial for bone health, immune function, and overall well-being.

Rich in Antioxidants: Mushrooms contain antioxidants, including ergothioneine and selenium, which help protect cells from damage caused by free radicals. Antioxidants play a role in supporting overall health and reducing the risk of chronic diseases.

Immune-Boosting Beta-Glucans: Beta-glucans, a type of soluble fiber found in mushrooms, have been linked to immune system modulation. They may enhance the activity of certain immune cells, contributing to a strengthened defense against infections.

Gut Health Support: Mushrooms are a good source of prebiotics, which nourish beneficial gut bacteria. A healthy gut microbiome is associated with various aspects of well-being, including digestion and immune function.

Different Varieties and Flavors: Each mushroom variety brings its own unique flavor profile to dishes. Shiitake mushrooms have a savory and smoky taste, while chanterelles offer a fruity, peppery note. The earthy flavor of porcini mushrooms and the delicate taste of oyster mushrooms add depth to culinary creations.

Umami Sensation: Mushrooms are known for their umami, the fifth basic taste that imparts a savory, satisfying quality to foods. This makes them an excellent addition to vegetarian and vegan dishes, providing depth and richness.

Medicinal Uses: Certain mushrooms, such as reishi and maitake, have been used in traditional medicine for their potential health benefits. These mushrooms are often available in supplement form and may have immune-modulating and anti-inflammatory properties.

Sustainable Farming: Mushrooms are known for their efficient use of resources in farming. They can be cultivated indoors, year-round, using organic waste materials, making them a sustainable and environmentally friendly crop.

Conclusion:

Mushrooms, with their diverse flavors, textures, and nutritional benefits, have carved a niche as a culinary and nutritional treasure. From adding depth to savory dishes to providing essential nutrients and potential health benefits, mushrooms continue to captivate taste buds and contribute to the rich tapestry of global cuisine. Whether enjoyed in a hearty stew, a gourmet pizza, or a simple stir-fry, mushrooms stand as earthy delights that bring both gastronomic pleasure and nourishment to the table.

Nectarines

Nectarines, the smooth-skinned cousins of peaches, are a delectable summer delight cherished for their juicy, sweet flavor and vibrant colors. These stone fruits not only offer a refreshing treat on a hot day but also pack a nutritional punch. Let's explore the characteristics, nutritional benefits, and culinary versatility that make nectarines a beloved addition to the summer fruit basket.

Succulent Sweetness: Nectarines are renowned for their juicy, sweet taste. Their flesh can range from white to yellow, and the flavor profile can vary from mildly sweet to intensely fruity, depending on the variety.

Nutrient-Rich Goodness: Nectarines are not only delicious but also provide essential nutrients. A one-cup serving (about 150 grams) of sliced nectarines offers approximately:

  - Calories: 62

  - Vitamin C: 14% of the Recommended Daily Allowance (RDA)

- Vitamin A: 7% of the RDA

- Dietary Fiber: 2.4 grams

- Potassium: 5% of the RDA

- Antioxidants: Including beta-carotene and flavonoids.

Hydration Boost: With their high water content, nectarines contribute to hydration, making them a refreshing choice during the warm summer months. Staying hydrated is essential for overall health and well-being.

Rich in Antioxidants: Nectarines contain antioxidants such as beta-carotene and quercetin, which help combat oxidative stress and inflammation in the body. Antioxidants play a role in maintaining cellular health.

Support for Skin Health: The vitamin C content in nectarines is beneficial for skin health, as it supports collagen synthesis, which contributes to the elasticity and firmness of the skin.

Dietary Fiber for Digestive Health: Nectarines provide dietary fiber, promoting digestive health by supporting regular bowel movements and aiding in the prevention of constipation.

Culinary Versatility: Nectarines shine in a variety of culinary applications. Some popular ways to enjoy nectarines include:

- Fresh and Raw: Sliced or bitten into as a refreshing snack.

- Salads: Added to green salads or fruit salads for a burst of sweetness.

- Smoothies: Blended into smoothies for a naturally sweet and creamy texture.

- Grilled or Roasted: Enhances the natural sugars and brings a caramelized flavor to desserts, main dishes, or side dishes.

Seasonal Delight: Nectarines are at their peak during the summer season, making them a highly anticipated and cherished fruit during warm weather. Their availability adds a burst of color and flavor to farmers' markets and grocery stores.

Varieties for Every Palate: There are various nectarine varieties, each with its unique characteristics. Some are freestone, meaning the flesh easily separates from the pit, while others are clingstone. Yellow and white nectarines offer different flavor profiles, allowing consumers to choose based on personal preference.

Pairing with Other Fruits: Nectarines complement a wide range of fruits in both sweet and savory dishes. They pair well with berries, citrus fruits, melons, and even savory ingredients like goat cheese and prosciutto in salads.

Conclusion:

Nectarines, with their succulent sweetness and nutritional richness, embody the essence of summer in every bite. Whether enjoyed fresh, grilled, or blended into a refreshing beverage, these stone fruits contribute to the sensory delights of the season. Beyond their delicious taste, nectarines offer a nutritious boost, making them a wholesome choice for those seeking both flavor and health benefits in their summer fruit selections.

Okra

Okra, also known as ladyfinger or gumbo, is a green, seed-filled pod that is both a culinary delight and a nutritional powerhouse. Loved for its unique texture and ability to enhance a variety of dishes, okra is a staple in many cuisines around the world. Let's explore the characteristics, nutritional benefits, and culinary versatility that make okra a standout ingredient in the realm of vegetables.

Distinctive Appearance and Texture: Okra pods are typically long and slender, with a ridged surface. When sliced, okra releases a mucilaginous substance, which gives it a unique, slightly slimy texture when cooked. This mucilage is valued for its thickening properties in soups and stews.

Nutrient-Rich Composition: Okra is a low-calorie vegetable that provides an array of essential nutrients. A one-cup serving (about 100 grams) of raw okra contains approximately:

- Calories: 33

- Protein: 1.9 grams

- Dietary Fiber: 3.2 grams

- Vitamin C: 23% of the Recommended Daily Allowance (RDA)

- Vitamin K: 31% of the RDA

- Folate (Vitamin B9): 15% of the RDA

- Magnesium: 14% of the RDA

Rich in Antioxidants: Okra is a good source of antioxidants, including flavonoids and polyphenols. These compounds help neutralize free radicals in the body, contributing to overall health and well-being.

Digestive Health Benefits: The mucilage in okra has a lubricating effect on the digestive tract, potentially aiding in the prevention of constipation. Additionally, the fiber content supports a healthy digestive system.

Heart-Healthy Nutrients: Okra contains potassium, a mineral that helps regulate blood pressure. The combination of potassium and fiber contributes to heart health by supporting optimal cardiovascular function.

Blood Sugar Regulation: The fiber content in okra may help regulate blood sugar levels by slowing the absorption of sugar in the digestive tract. This can be beneficial for individuals with diabetes or those at risk of developing the condition.

Culinary Versatility: Okra is incredibly versatile in the kitchen and can be prepared in various ways. Some popular cooking methods include:

- Sautéed or Stir-Fried: Enhances the natural flavor and reduces sliminess.

- Grilled or Roasted: Develops a smoky flavor and crispy texture.

- Stewed or Braised: Well-suited for soups, stews, and gumbo dishes.

- Pickled: Preserves okra while adding a tangy flavor.

Global Culinary Presence: Okra is a key ingredient in many global cuisines, particularly in Southern United States cuisine, Middle Eastern dishes, Indian curries, and African stews. Its adaptability and ability to complement various flavors make it a favorite in diverse culinary traditions.

Seasonal Availability: Okra is typically in season during the warmer months, making it a fresh and seasonal addition to summer and early fall dishes.

Gardening and Growing Okra: Okra plants are relatively easy to grow in warm climates. They thrive in well-drained soil and sunny conditions. Home gardeners often enjoy cultivating okra for its prolific production.

Conclusion:

Okra, with its distinctive texture and nutritional richness, stands as a versatile and healthful addition to a variety of dishes. Whether enjoyed in savory stews, pickled snacks, or crispy stir-fries, okra invites culinary creativity and contributes to a well-balanced diet. Beyond its culinary merits, okra brings a host of potential health benefits, making it a valued ingredient in kitchens around the world.

Onions

Onions, with their pungent aroma and distinctive flavor, are a fundamental ingredient in kitchens worldwide. These versatile bulbs belong to the Allium family and come in various types, each offering a unique taste profile. Beyond their culinary significance, onions boast health benefits and have been used for centuries for both culinary and medicinal purposes. Let's delve into the characteristics, nutritional value, and culinary versatility that make onions a kitchen staple.

Diverse Varieties: Onions come in various types, each with its flavor intensity and preferred culinary use. Common varieties include:

- Yellow Onions: Versatile and widely used in savory dishes.

- Red Onions: Mild and slightly sweet, often used raw in salads.

- White Onions: Crisp and sharp, suitable for Mexican and Southwestern cuisines.

- Sweet Onions (e.g., Vidalia, Walla Walla): Mild and less pungent, excellent for salads and grilling.

- Shallots: Small, mild bulbs with a subtle garlic flavor, popular in French cuisine.

Nutritional Value: Onions are low in calories but rich in essential nutrients. A one-cup (about 160 grams) serving of chopped onions provides approximately:

- Calories: 64

- Fiber: 3.0 grams

- Vitamin C: 16% of the Recommended Daily Allowance (RDA)

- Folate (Vitamin B9): 8% of the RDA

- Potassium: 7% of the RDA

- Manganese: 7% of the RDA

- Vitamin B6: 6% of the RDA

Antioxidant and Anti-Inflammatory Properties: Onions contain antioxidants, including quercetin, which has anti-inflammatory and immune-boosting properties. These compounds may contribute to overall health and help combat oxidative stress.

Heart Health Benefits: The sulfur compounds in onions may have cardiovascular benefits, including the potential to lower blood pressure and reduce the risk of heart disease. The presence of quercetin may also contribute to heart health.

Immune Support: Vitamin C, found in onions, is crucial for immune function, helping the body defend against infections and illnesses.

Culinary Versatility: Onions serve as a foundation for countless savory dishes, imparting depth and complexity of flavor. They can be prepared in various ways, such as:

- Sautéed: Enhances the natural sweetness and softens the texture.

- Caramelized: Develops a rich, sweet flavor, ideal for topping burgers or adding to soups.

- Raw: Adds a crisp, pungent kick to salads, salsas, and sandwiches.

- Pickled: Offers a tangy, zesty element to dishes.

Essential in Global Cuisines: Onions are a staple in cuisines around the world, playing a central role in the flavor profiles of dishes from Italian pasta sauces to Indian curries. They are often part of the culinary "holy trinity" or "sofrito" in various regional cooking traditions.

Medicinal Uses: Onions have been used historically for their potential medicinal properties. They were valued for their antibacterial and antifungal effects and were applied topically to wounds or consumed to promote overall health.

Storage and Longevity: Onions have a relatively long shelf life and can be stored in a cool, dry place. Properly stored onions can last for several weeks to months, making them a convenient pantry staple.

Culinary Companion: Onions are often paired with garlic, creating a dynamic duo that forms the base of many savory dishes. Together, they contribute to the complex and layered flavors that characterize a wide range of cuisines.

Conclusion:

Onions, with their aromatic allure and culinary prowess, are essential ingredients that add depth and character to countless dishes. From enhancing the savory goodness of soups to providing a crisp bite in salads, onions are culinary companions that transcend cultural boundaries. Beyond their culinary contributions, the health benefits and historical significance of onions underscore their role as both a kitchen staple and a symbol of flavorful abundance.

Oranges

Oranges, the vibrant and refreshing citrus fruits, are celebrated not only for their sweet and tangy flavor but also for their nutritional richness. Whether enjoyed fresh, juiced, or incorporated into various culinary creations, oranges are a delightful source of essential vitamins, minerals, and antioxidants. Let's explore the characteristics, nutritional benefits, and versatile uses that make oranges a beloved fruit worldwide.

Citrus Brilliance: Oranges belong to the citrus genus, known for their bright colors, juicy pulp, and characteristic citrus aroma. They come in various varieties, including navel oranges, Valencia oranges, blood oranges, and mandarins, each with its unique taste and appearance.

Vitamin C Powerhouse: Oranges are renowned for their exceptionally high vitamin C content. A medium-sized orange (about 131 grams) provides approximately:

- Calories: 62

- Vitamin C: 70% of the Recommended Daily Allowance (RDA)

- Fiber: 3.1 grams

- Potassium: 6% of the RDA

- Vitamin A: 4% of the RDA

Immune System Support: Vitamin C is a potent antioxidant that plays a crucial role in supporting the immune system. It helps stimulate the production of white blood cells and protects cells from oxidative stress.

Fiber for Digestive Health: Oranges are a good source of dietary fiber, particularly soluble fiber known as pectin. Fiber supports digestive health by promoting regular bowel movements and aiding in the prevention of constipation.

Antioxidant Properties: Oranges contain various antioxidants, including flavonoids and carotenoids, which help neutralize free radicals. Antioxidants contribute to overall health and may reduce the risk of chronic diseases.

Heart Health Benefits: Potassium, present in oranges, is essential for heart health. It helps regulate blood pressure and supports proper cardiovascular function.

Hydration and Refreshment: With their high water content, oranges contribute to hydration, making them a juicy and refreshing snack, especially in warm weather.

Culinary Versatility: Oranges are incredibly versatile in the kitchen. Some popular uses include:

- Fresh and Juiced: Enjoyed as a standalone snack or squeezed into refreshing orange juice.

- Salads: Added to fruit salads or green salads for a burst of sweetness.

- Desserts: Featured in cakes, sorbets, and tarts for a citrusy twist.

- Sauces and Marinades: Used to enhance the flavor of savory dishes, especially in Asian and Mediterranean cuisines.

Seasonal Cheer: Oranges are often associated with the winter season, where they bring a burst of color and freshness to holiday celebrations. Citrus fruits, including oranges, are a classic addition to festive displays.

Symbolic Significance: Oranges have symbolic significance in various cultures. They are associated with good luck, prosperity, and abundance in some traditions and are often exchanged during festive occasions.

Conclusion:

Oranges, with their juicy sweetness and nutritional richness, stand as iconic symbols of health and refreshment. Whether savored in their natural form, juiced, or incorporated into a variety of dishes, oranges contribute to a well-balanced and flavorful diet. Beyond their culinary appeal, the vitamin C-packed citrus fruits serve as a reminder of the vibrant and nourishing qualities that nature offers, making them a cherished addition to the global repertoire of fruits.

Papaya

Papaya, often referred to as the "fruit of angels," is a tropical delight known for its vibrant color, sweet taste, and abundance of health benefits. This tropical fruit is not only delicious but also rich in essential vitamins, enzymes, and antioxidants. Let's explore the characteristics, nutritional value, and health-promoting qualities that make papaya a popular and nutritious addition to the fruit basket.

Tropical Splendor: Papaya, with its elongated shape and orange flesh, is a tropical fruit that thrives in warm climates. The ripe fruit has a sweet and succulent flavor, making it a refreshing treat, especially during hot weather.

Nutrient-Rich Composition: Papaya is a nutritional powerhouse, providing an array of essential nutrients in a low-calorie package. A one-cup (about 140 grams) serving of papaya offers approximately:

- Calories: 59

- Vitamin C: 88% of the Recommended Daily Allowance (RDA)

- Vitamin A: 33% of the RDA

- Fiber: 3 grams

- Folate (Vitamin B9): 14% of the RDA

- Potassium: 11% of the RDA

- Enzymes (Papain): Aids in digestion

Digestive Enzymes: Papaya contains an enzyme called papain, which aids in the digestion of proteins. This makes papaya a digestive-friendly fruit and has led to its use in traditional medicine for digestive support.

Rich in Antioxidants: Papaya is loaded with antioxidants, including beta-carotene, lutein, and zeaxanthin. These compounds help neutralize free radicals, offering potential protection against oxidative stress and inflammation.

Immune Support: The high vitamin C content in papaya supports the immune system by promoting the production of white blood cells and enhancing the body's ability to fight infections.

Heart-Healthy Nutrients: Potassium in papaya contributes to heart health by helping regulate blood pressure. The fiber content also aids in maintaining healthy cholesterol levels.

Skin Health Benefits: The combination of vitamins A, C, and E in papaya, along with its antioxidant content, is beneficial for skin health. These nutrients may contribute to a healthy complexion and protect the skin from premature aging.

Culinary Versatility: Papaya is a versatile fruit that can be enjoyed in various ways. Some popular uses include:

- Fresh and Sliced: As a standalone snack or part of fruit salads.

- Smoothies: Blended into refreshing beverages for a tropical twist.

- Salsas: Combined with other fruits, vegetables, and herbs for a sweet and tangy salsa.

- Desserts: Featured in sorbets, ice creams, and fruity desserts.

Papaya Seeds: While the focus is often on the sweet flesh, papaya seeds are edible and have a peppery flavor. They are sometimes used as a seasoning or incorporated into dressings.

Tropical Symbolism: Papaya is often associated with tropical paradises and is a symbol of abundance and vitality in various cultures. Its bright color and tropical charm make it a favorite in exotic destinations.

Conclusion:

Papaya, with its tropical sweetness and nutritional richness, stands as a testament to the bountiful offerings of the natural world. Whether enjoyed fresh, blended into beverages, or used to enhance culinary creations, papaya brings a burst of flavor and nourishment. As a versatile and health-promoting fruit, papaya continues to be celebrated not only for its delicious taste but also for the vibrant energy it brings to the tropical tapestry of fruits.

Peaches

Peaches, the succulent and fragrant fruits, are synonymous with the warmth of summer and are cherished for their sweet, velvety flesh. Whether enjoyed fresh, grilled, or transformed into various culinary delights, peaches are a true embodiment of the season's bounty. Let's explore the characteristics, nutritional benefits, and culinary versatility that make peaches a beloved and delectable fruit.

Velvety Goodness: Peaches are recognized by their fuzzy, velvety skin, which conceals the tender, juicy flesh within. They come in various varieties, including clingstone and freestone, with colors ranging from yellow to blush.

Nutrient-Rich Profile: Peaches offer a range of essential nutrients while being relatively low in calories. A one-cup (about 154 grams) serving of sliced peaches provides approximately:

- Calories: 60

- Vitamin C: 11% of the Recommended Daily Allowance (RDA)

- Vitamin A: 10% of the RDA

- Dietary Fiber: 2 grams

- Potassium: 8% of the RDA

- Antioxidants: Including beta-carotene and lutein.

Antioxidant Richness: Peaches are rich in antioxidants, which help combat oxidative stress and inflammation in the body. The presence of carotenoids and flavonoids contributes to their potential health benefits.

Hydration and Refreshment: With their high water content, peaches contribute to hydration, making them a refreshing and juicy snack on hot summer days.

Fiber for Digestive Health: Peaches contain dietary fiber, which supports digestive health by promoting regular bowel movements and aiding in the prevention of constipation.

Heart-Healthy Potassium: Potassium in peaches plays a role in maintaining healthy blood pressure levels and supporting overall cardiovascular health.

Culinary Versatility: Peaches are incredibly versatile in the kitchen and can be enjoyed in a variety of ways. Some popular culinary uses include:

- Fresh and Juicy: Eaten as a standalone fruit or added to fruit salads.

- Grilled: Enhances the natural sweetness and adds a smoky flavor.

- Desserts: Featured in pies, cobblers, crisps, and ice creams.

- Preserves and Jams: Used to create sweet spreads for toast or desserts.

- Salsas: Combined with herbs and spices for a delightful accompaniment to savory dishes.

Seasonal Delight: Peaches are at their peak during the summer months, and their availability marks the height of the season's fruitfulness. Local peach orchards and farmers' markets showcase the diversity of peach varieties.

Symbolic Significance: Peaches have symbolic significance in various cultures, often representing fertility, longevity, and sweetness. They are associated with positive attributes and are sometimes featured in cultural rituals and traditions.

Orchard Beauty: The experience of picking peaches from an orchard adds to the charm of these fruits. Many regions host peach-picking events, allowing people to connect with the source of this seasonal delight.

Conclusion:

Peaches, with their juicy sweetness and versatility, capture the essence of summer's bounty. Whether enjoyed in their natural state, incorporated into desserts, or featured in savory dishes, peaches bring joy and flavor to the table. As a symbol of warmth and abundance, peaches continue to be a favorite fruit, inviting everyone to savor the fleeting moments of summer sweetness.

Pears

Pears, characterized by their elegant shape and smooth skin, are not only visually appealing but also offer a delightful combination of juiciness and subtle sweetness. These versatile fruits come in various varieties, each with its unique flavor profile, making them a favorite for both snacking and culinary creations. Let's explore the characteristics, nutritional benefits, and culinary versatility that make pears a timeless and beloved fruit.

Elegant Varieties: Pears come in diverse varieties, including Anjou, Bartlett, Bosc, Comice, and Asian pears. Each variety has its own texture, flavor, and color, ranging from the classic green and red to the distinctive golden-brown.

Nutrient-Rich Goodness: Pears are not only delicious but also pack a nutritional punch. A one-cup (about 185 grams) serving of sliced pears provides approximately:

- Calories: 100

- Dietary Fiber: 6 grams

- Vitamin C: 12% of the Recommended Daily Allowance (RDA)

- Potassium: 4% of the RDA

- Copper: 4% of the RDA

- Vitamin K: 6% of the RDA

Rich in Dietary Fiber: Pears are an excellent source of dietary fiber, particularly soluble fiber known as pectin. This fiber supports digestive health, aids in weight management, and helps regulate blood sugar levels.

Antioxidant Content: Pears contain antioxidants, including vitamin C and various phytochemicals, which help neutralize free radicals. Antioxidants play a role in promoting overall health and reducing the risk of chronic diseases.

Hydration and Low Calories: With their high water content and relatively low calorie count, pears contribute to hydration while making a satisfying and healthy snack option.

Heart-Healthy Potassium: Pears contain potassium, an essential mineral that supports heart health by helping regulate blood pressure and promoting cardiovascular function.

Culinary Versatility: Pears lend themselves to a variety of culinary applications. Some popular ways to enjoy pears include:

- Fresh and Raw: As a juicy snack or sliced in salads.

- Poached: Infused with spices and sweeteners for an elegant dessert.

- Baked or Grilled: Enhances the natural sweetness and adds a caramelized flavor.

- Preserves and Jams: Used to create sweet spreads for toast or pastries.

- In Desserts: Featured in tarts, crisps, and pies for a delightful fruity addition.

Seasonal Abundance: Pears are often associated with the fall season, where their availability adds to the richness of autumn harvests. Local farmers' markets showcase a variety of pears, inviting consumers to explore different flavors.

Pairing with Cheese: Pears pair exceptionally well with various cheeses, creating a classic and sophisticated combination enjoyed in cheese platters and gourmet dishes.

Symbol of Longevity: In various cultures, pears symbolize longevity, good health, and prosperity. The fruit's association with these positive attributes adds to its cultural significance.

Conclusion:

Pears, with their elegant appearance and balanced sweetness, stand as a testament to the diversity of nature's offerings. Whether enjoyed fresh, baked into delectable desserts, or paired with cheeses, pears bring a touch of sophistication and natural sweetness to the table. As a symbol of seasonal abundance and culinary versatility, pears continue to be a timeless and cherished fruit enjoyed in various forms around the world.

Peppers

Peppers, encompassing a diverse family of both sweet bell peppers and fiery chili peppers, are culinary gems that add vibrancy and depth to dishes around the world. Whether bringing a burst of sweetness to salads or infusing heat into spicy cuisines, peppers contribute a dynamic spectrum of flavors and nutritional benefits. Let's explore the characteristics, nutritional value, and culinary versatility that make peppers an essential and exciting part of the global culinary landscape.

Sweet Bell Peppers:

- Varieties and Colors: Bell peppers come in an array of colors, including green, red, yellow, orange, and even purple. Each color has its own distinct flavor profile, with red peppers generally being sweeter and green peppers having a slightly bitter taste.

- Flavor Profile: Sweet bell peppers contribute a mild, crisp sweetness to dishes, making them versatile in various culinary applications.

Chili Peppers:

- Varieties and Heat Levels: Chili peppers, on the other hand, vary widely in heat levels. From the mild poblano to the fiery habanero, chili peppers add varying degrees of spiciness to dishes.

- Scoville Scale: The Scoville Heat Scale measures the heat intensity of chili peppers. For example, bell peppers rate at 0 Scoville Heat Units (SHU), while a habanero can exceed 350,000 SHU.

Nutritional Value:

- Vitamins and Minerals: Peppers are rich in essential nutrients. A one-cup (about 149 grams) serving of chopped bell peppers provides approximately:

  - Calories: 46

  - Vitamin C: 211% of the Recommended Daily Allowance (RDA)

  - Vitamin A: 44% of the RDA

  - Fiber: 3 grams

  - Potassium: 6% of the RDA

Antioxidant-Rich:

- Vitamins A and C: The high levels of vitamins A and C in peppers act as antioxidants, helping protect cells from damage caused by free radicals.

Capsaicin and Health Benefits:

- Chili Peppers: The compound responsible for the heat in chili peppers, capsaicin, has been linked to various health benefits. It may aid in weight management, boost metabolism, and even have anti-inflammatory properties.

Culinary Versatility:

- Raw and Crunchy: Bell peppers are delightful when sliced and added to salads or enjoyed as crunchy snacks.

- Grilled or Roasted: Enhances the natural sweetness and imparts a smoky flavor.

- Stuffed: Bell peppers are often stuffed with a variety of ingredients, creating a satisfying and visually appealing dish.

- Salsas and Hot Sauces: Chili peppers are key ingredients in salsas and hot sauces, adding heat and depth to the flavors.

- Curries and Stir-Fries: Chili peppers are central to many cuisines, providing the characteristic spiciness to dishes like Thai curries and Sichuan stir-fries.

Global Culinary Influence:

- Mediterranean Cuisine: Bell peppers are integral to Mediterranean dishes, such as stuffed peppers and ratatouille.

- Mexican and Thai Cuisine: Chili peppers play a central role in the spiciness of Mexican salsas and Thai curries.

- Indian Cuisine: Chili peppers are essential in various forms in Indian cuisine, from the milder green chilies to the intensely hot ghost peppers.

Preserving Peppers:

- Drying: Chili peppers can be dried and ground into powders, preserving their heat and flavor.

- Pickling: Both sweet and hot peppers can be pickled, providing a tangy and spicy condiment.

Gardening Appeal:

- Home Cultivation: Peppers are popular choices for home gardens due to their adaptability and the satisfaction of growing fresh produce.

Cultural Symbolism:

- Mild and Fiery Symbolism: In various cultures, the contrast between sweet bell peppers and hot chili peppers symbolizes the spectrum of flavors in life, from the mild to the fiery.

Conclusion:

Peppers, with their diverse flavors and heat levels, contribute an exciting and colorful dimension to the world of cuisine. Whether adding a pop of sweetness or a kick of spice, peppers play a crucial role in enhancing the depth and complexity of dishes across cultures. From mild to hot, these culinary wonders continue to captivate taste buds and elevate the global palate.

Pineapple

Pineapple, with its tropical allure and distinctively sweet flavor, is a fruit that brings a taste of paradise to any dish. Whether enjoyed fresh, juiced, grilled, or incorporated into various culinary creations, pineapple is celebrated for its refreshing and vibrant qualities. Let's explore the characteristics, nutritional benefits, and culinary versatility that make pineapple a favorite among fruits.

Tropical Splendor:

- Appearance: Pineapple is instantly recognizable with its spiky, rough exterior and crown of leaves.

- Flavor Profile: Known for its sweet and tangy taste, pineapple adds a refreshing burst of flavor.

Nutrient-Rich Goodness:

- Vitamins and Minerals: A one-cup (about 165 grams) serving of pineapple provides approximately:

  - Calories: 82

  - Vitamin C: 131% of the Recommended Daily Allowance (RDA)

  - Manganese: 76% of the RDA

  - Dietary Fiber: 2.3 grams

  - Vitamin B6: 9% of the RDA

Enzyme Bromelain:

- Digestive Aid: Pineapple contains bromelain, an enzyme with anti-inflammatory properties that may aid in digestion and reduce bloating.

Antioxidant Richness:

- Vitamin C: The high vitamin C content in pineapple acts as an antioxidant, helping to protect cells from damage caused by free radicals.

Hydration and Low Calories:

- Water Content: With its high water content, pineapple contributes to hydration.

- Calorie-Friendly: Pineapple is relatively low in calories, making it a guilt-free and satisfying snack.

Culinary Versatility:

- Fresh and Juicy: Enjoyed as a standalone snack or added to fruit salads.

- Smoothies and Juices: Blended into tropical beverages for a refreshing treat.

- Grilled or Roasted: Develops a caramelized flavor, perfect for desserts or savory dishes.

- Salsas and Chutneys: Adds sweetness and acidity to complement savory dishes.

- Desserts: Featured in cakes, sorbets, and tarts for a delightful tropical twist.

Seasonal Allure:

- Summer Staple: Pineapple is often associated with summertime, where its availability adds a tropical touch to seasonal dishes and beverages.

Symbolic Significance:

- Hospitality: In some cultures, pineapple is a symbol of hospitality and welcome, making it a popular choice in hospitality industry logos and decorations.

Dried Pineapple:

- Snack Option: Dried pineapple is a convenient and sweet snack, retaining the fruit's natural sweetness in a chewy form.

Pineapple Expressions:

- Expressive Shapes: Pineapple's distinctive appearance has inspired art, decor, and fashion, making it a symbol of playful expression.

Conclusion:

Pineapple, with its tropical charm and nutritional richness, is more than just a fruit—it's a symbol of sunshine and delight. Whether savored fresh, blended into beverages, or incorporated into a variety of dishes, pineapple brings a burst of sweetness and vibrancy to the palate. As a versatile and refreshing fruit, pineapple continues to be a tropical treasure enjoyed globally, bringing a taste of the exotic to tables around the world.

Plums

Plums, with their succulent flesh and smooth skin, are a quintessential fruit of the summer season. Bursting with sweetness and a delightful tartness, plums come in an array of colors and varieties, making them a versatile and refreshing addition to both sweet and savory dishes. Let's explore the characteristics, nutritional benefits, and culinary versatility that make plums a cherished and delicious fruit.

Variety of Colors: Plums come in a spectrum of colors, including red, purple, yellow, and green. The skin can be smooth or slightly tart, while the flesh ranges from firm to exceptionally juicy.

Nutrient-Rich Profile: A one-cup (about 165 grams) serving of sliced plums provides approximately:

- Calories: 76

- Vitamin C: 26% of the Recommended Daily Allowance (RDA)

- Vitamin K: 24% of the RDA

- Dietary Fiber: 3 grams

- Potassium: 8% of the RDA

Antioxidant Richness: Plums are rich in antioxidants, including phenolic compounds, which contribute to their vibrant colors and potential health benefits.

Heart-Healthy Potassium: Plums contain potassium, a mineral essential for maintaining healthy blood pressure and supporting cardiovascular health.

Digestive Support: Plums are a good source of dietary fiber, promoting digestive health and contributing to regular bowel movements.

Culinary Versatility:

- Fresh and Ripe: Enjoyed as a juicy and refreshing snack, or added to fruit salads.

- Preserves and Jams: Used to create sweet spreads for toast, pastries, or as an accompaniment to savory dishes.

- Desserts: Featured in pies, tarts, crisps, and ice creams for a burst of natural sweetness.

- Savory Dishes: Plums can be incorporated into savory dishes, adding a touch of sweetness to sauces, chutneys, and meat marinades.

Dried Plums (Prunes):

- Nutrient Concentration: Dried plums, commonly known as prunes, are a concentrated source of nutrients, including fiber, potassium, and certain vitamins.

- Digestive Health: Prunes are often associated with digestive health, known for their natural laxative properties.

Seasonal Beauty: Plums are at their peak during the summer months, contributing to the bounty of seasonal fruits.

Cultural Significance: In various cultures, plums symbolize different qualities, including good fortune, abundance, and sweetness.

Orchard Pleasures: Many regions offer the joy of picking plums directly from orchards, allowing people to experience the freshness and variety of this summer fruit.

Conclusion:

Plums, with their juicy sweetness and vibrant colors, capture the essence of summer's abundance. Whether savored fresh, dried as prunes, or incorporated into a variety of dishes, plums bring a burst of flavor and nutritional goodness to the table. As a symbol of seasonal delight and culinary versatility, plums continue to be a cherished fruit enjoyed in various forms around the world.

Pomegranates

Pomegranates, often hailed as the "jewels of antiquity," are fruits that have graced tables and cultural narratives for centuries. Known for their ruby-red arils and rich, slightly tart flavor, pomegranates are not just a delicious treat but also a symbol of health, fertility, and prosperity. Let's explore the characteristics, nutritional benefits, and cultural significance that make pomegranates a unique and celebrated fruit.

Ancient Symbolism: Pomegranates have symbolic importance in various cultures, representing fertility, abundance, and prosperity. They are often featured in art, literature, and religious symbolism.

Ruby-Red Arils: Pomegranates are characterized by their tough outer rind, concealing clusters of juicy, jewel-like arils. Each aril contains a seed surrounded by a translucent, sweet, and slightly tart pulp.

Nutrient-Rich Profile: A one-cup (about 174 grams) serving of arils provides approximately:

- Calories: 83

- Vitamin C: 28% of the Recommended Daily Allowance (RDA)

- Vitamin K: 24% of the RDA

- Fiber: 4 grams

- Folate (Vitamin B9): 10% of the RDA

- Antioxidants: Including punicalagins and anthocyanins.

Heart-Healthy Properties: Pomegranates contain potent antioxidants that may contribute to heart health by reducing oxidative stress and inflammation.

Anti-Inflammatory Potential: Pomegranates are rich in polyphenols, which have been studied for their potential anti-inflammatory effects.

Digestive Health: Pomegranates are a good source of dietary fiber, supporting digestive health and contributing to regular bowel movements.

Culinary Versatility:

- Fresh and Raw: Arils can be enjoyed as a refreshing snack or added to fruit salads.

- Juiced: Pomegranate juice is popular for its sweet and tangy flavor, often used in beverages, cocktails, and culinary creations.

- Seeds in Savory Dishes: Pomegranate arils add a burst of sweetness to salads, yogurt, and various savory dishes.

- Sauces and Dressings: Pomegranate molasses, made from reduced pomegranate juice, is used to enhance the flavor of sauces and dressings.

Pomegranate Molasses: Pomegranate molasses is a versatile condiment with a sweet and tangy flavor, used in Middle Eastern and Mediterranean cuisines.

Seasonal Delight: Pomegranates are typically harvested in the fall, adding a burst of color and flavor to seasonal dishes.

Medicinal Uses: In some cultures, pomegranates have been used in traditional medicine for their perceived health benefits, including their potential role in supporting heart health and digestion.

Conclusion:

Pomegranates, with their rich history, vibrant appearance, and nutritional richness, continue to captivate both culinary enthusiasts and health-conscious individuals. Whether savored in their natural form, juiced, or incorporated into a variety of dishes, pomegranates bring a unique blend of sweetness and tartness to the table. As symbols of prosperity and vitality, these ancient jewels remain a cherished and flavorful addition to global culinary traditions.

Radishes

Radishes, with their vibrant colors, crisp texture, and distinct peppery flavor, are humble yet versatile root vegetables that add a refreshing crunch to salads, garnishes, and various culinary creations. Whether enjoyed raw or cooked, radishes bring a unique zest to the table. Let's explore the characteristics, nutritional benefits, and culinary versatility that make radishes a delightful addition to a diverse range of dishes.

Assorted Varieties: Radishes come in various shapes and colors, from the classic round red radishes to elongated daikon radishes in white or pale green. The watermelon radish, with its green exterior and pink interior, adds visual appeal to dishes.

Crisp and Refreshing: Radishes are prized for their crisp texture, providing a satisfying crunch that can elevate the overall eating experience.

- Peppery Flavor: The flavor of radishes ranges from mildly peppery to more assertive, depending on the variety.

Nutrient-Rich Profile: A one-cup (about 116 grams) serving of sliced radishes provides approximately:

- Calories: 19

- Vitamin C: 18% of the Recommended Daily Allowance (RDA)

- Folate (Vitamin B9): 3% of the RDA

- Potassium: 270 mg

- Fiber: 2 grams

Antioxidant Content: Radishes contain various phytochemicals with antioxidant properties, helping to neutralize free radicals in the body.

Digestive Health: Radishes contribute to digestive health by providing dietary fiber, supporting regular bowel movements and promoting a healthy gut.

Culinary Versatility:

- Raw in Salads: Sliced or shredded radishes add a peppery kick and vibrant color to salads.

- Pickled: Radishes are often pickled, offering a tangy and crunchy addition to sandwiches, tacos, or rice bowls.

- Roasted: Roasting radishes can mellow their sharpness, turning them into a savory side dish.

- Cooked in Soups or Stir-Fries: Daikon radishes are particularly popular in Asian cuisines, where they are used in soups, stews, and stir-fries.

Garnishes and Appetizers: Radishes can be intricately sliced to create decorative radish roses, often used as garnishes on platters and appetizers.

Daikon Radish in Sushi: Daikon radish is commonly used as a filling for sushi rolls, providing a crisp and mildly flavored contrast to other ingredients.

Growing Popularity: Radishes are favored by home gardeners for their quick growth, making them a popular choice in farm-to-table initiatives.

Low-Calorie Snack: With their low calorie count and high water content, radishes make for a refreshing and guilt-free snack.

Conclusion:

Radishes, with their refreshing crispness and peppery zing, bring a burst of flavor and color to the culinary landscape. From salads to pickles and a variety of cooked dishes, radishes showcase their versatility and add a delightful element to meals. As a garden gem that thrives in diversity, radishes continue to be a favorite for those seeking both flavor and nutritional value in their culinary adventures.

Raspberries

Raspberries, with their jewel-like appearance and luscious, sweet-tart flavor, are among the most beloved berries. These vibrant red gems are not only delightful to the taste buds but also pack a nutritional punch, making them a popular choice for fresh snacking, desserts, and a variety of culinary creations. Let's delve into the characteristics, nutritional benefits, and culinary versatility that make raspberries a delightful addition to the world of berries.

Jewel-Toned Beauty: Raspberries are small, delicate berries with a rich red hue and a cluster of drupelets that create a distinctive, jewel-like appearance.

Sweet-Tart Flavor: Raspberries offer a perfect balance of sweetness and tartness, making them a versatile ingredient in both sweet and savory dishes.

Nutrient-Rich Goodness: A one-cup (about 123 grams) serving of raspberries provides approximately:

- Calories: 64

- Dietary Fiber: 8 grams

- Vitamin C: 54% of the Recommended Daily Allowance (RDA)

- Manganese: 41% of the RDA

- Folate (Vitamin B9): 6% of the RDA

Antioxidant Power: Raspberries are rich in polyphenols and anthocyanins, antioxidants that contribute to their vibrant color and potential health benefits.

Heart-Healthy Fiber: The high fiber content in raspberries supports digestive health, helps regulate blood sugar levels, and contributes to heart health.

Anti-Inflammatory Properties: Raspberries contain quercetin, a flavonoid with anti-inflammatory properties that may contribute to overall health.

Culinary Versatility:

- Fresh and Simple: Enjoyed fresh as a snack or added to fruit salads for a burst of flavor.

- Desserts: Featured in pies, tarts, cakes, and ice creams, showcasing their natural sweetness.

- Smoothies: Blended into refreshing smoothies for a nutritious and delicious boost.

- Preserves and Jams: Used to create sweet spreads for breakfast or desserts.

- Savory Pairings: Raspberries can be paired with savory dishes, adding a unique touch to salads or incorporated into sauces for meat.

Seasonal Harvest: Raspberries are typically in peak season during the summer, adding a seasonal freshness to dishes.

Farm-to-Table Appeal: Raspberries are well-suited for home gardens, allowing enthusiasts to enjoy the pleasure of harvesting their own berries.

Symbol of Romance: Raspberries are often associated with romance and decadence, making them a popular choice for romantic desserts and celebrations.

Conclusion:

Raspberries, with their exquisite flavor and nutritional richness, stand as a testament to the diverse and delightful world of berries. Whether enjoyed fresh, incorporated into desserts, or used in creative culinary pairings, raspberries bring a burst of sweetness and vibrancy to the table. As jewels of the berry world, raspberries continue to be cherished for their culinary versatility, nutritional benefits, and irresistible charm.

Spinach

Spinach, with its dark green leaves and versatile culinary applications, is a leafy green that has earned its reputation as a nutrient powerhouse. Packed with vitamins, minerals, and antioxidants, spinach is not only a versatile ingredient in a variety of dishes but also a key player in promoting overall health. Let's explore the characteristics, nutritional benefits, and culinary versatility that make spinach a standout leafy green in the world of vegetables.

Leafy Green Goodness: Spinach has vibrant green, tender leaves that can be either smooth or slightly crinkled, depending on the variety.

Nutrient-Rich Profile: A one-cup (about 30 grams) serving of raw spinach provides approximately:

- Calories: 7

- Vitamin A: 188% of the Recommended Daily Allowance (RDA)

- Vitamin K: 460% of the RDA

- Folate (Vitamin B9): 49% of the RDA

- Iron: 15% of the RDA

- Calcium: 3% of the RDA

Antioxidant Power:

- Lutein and Zeaxanthin: Spinach contains these antioxidants, which are beneficial for eye health.

- Vitamin C and E: Spinach contributes to the body's antioxidant defense system.

Iron Source: While the iron in spinach is non-heme iron (plant-based), consuming it with vitamin C-rich foods can enhance iron absorption.

Heart-Healthy Nutrients: Spinach contains potassium, a mineral that supports heart health by helping regulate blood pressure.

Bone Health: Essential for bone health, spinach is a rich source of vitamin K, contributing to bone mineralization and density.

Fiber for Digestive Health: Spinach is a good source of fiber, promoting digestive health and aiding in weight management.

Culinary Versatility:

- Fresh in Salads: Enjoyed raw in salads, providing a refreshing and nutritious base.

- Cooked in Dishes: Added to sautés, soups, stews, and casseroles for a nutrient boost.

- Smoothies: Blended into smoothies for a nutrient-packed green addition.

- Stuffed Dishes: Used as a filling for stuffed chicken, pasta, or vegetarian dishes.

Baby Spinach: Baby spinach, with its tender leaves, is a popular choice for salads and quick sautés.

Easy to Grow: Spinach is relatively easy to grow, making it a favorite among home gardeners for its accessibility and nutritional value.

Conclusion:

Spinach, with its impressive nutrient profile and culinary versatility, rightfully earns its place as a nutritional powerhouse in the world of leafy greens. Whether enjoyed fresh, cooked, or blended into various dishes, spinach stands as a testament to the importance of incorporating nutrient-rich greens into a balanced diet. As a symbol of health and vitality, spinach continues to be a staple in kitchens and gardens, contributing both flavor and nutritional benefits to meals around the world.

Squash

Squash, a diverse and colorful family of vegetables, is a culinary gem that adds flavor, texture, and nutritional value to a variety of dishes. From summer squashes like zucchini to winter squashes like butternut, each variety brings its own unique qualities to the table. Let's explore the characteristics, nutritional benefits, and culinary versatility that make squash a standout ingredient in the world of vegetables.

Diverse Varieties:

- Summer Squashes: Varieties like zucchini and yellow squash are tender and mild, often enjoyed in their youthful state.

- Winter Squashes: Butternut, acorn, and spaghetti squashes are heartier, with a sweeter flavor, and are typically harvested in the mature stage.

Nutrient-Rich Goodness: A one-cup (about 205 grams) serving of cooked squash provides approximately:

- Calories: 42

- Vitamin A: 457% of the Recommended Daily Allowance (RDA)

- Vitamin C: 28% of the RDA

- Potassium: 13% of the RDA

- Fiber: 2.6 grams

Antioxidant Content: Squashes, particularly those with vibrant orange flesh, are rich in beta-carotene, a precursor to vitamin A with antioxidant properties.

Heart-Healthy Potassium: Squash contributes to heart health by providing potassium, which helps regulate blood pressure.

Dietary Fiber for Digestive Health: Squash is a good source of dietary fiber, supporting digestive health and promoting a feeling of fullness.

Low-Calorie Option: Squash is relatively low in calories, making it a nutritious and satisfying option for those watching their calorie intake.

Culinary Versatility:

- Roasted and Grilled: Enhances the natural sweetness and caramelizes the edges for a delicious side dish.

- Pureed: Used in soups, sauces, and baby food for a smooth and creamy texture.

- Sliced in Salads: Summer squashes, when thinly sliced, add a crisp texture to salads.

- Stuffed or Baked: Hollowed-out squashes can be filled with various ingredients, creating a hearty and flavorful dish.

- Spiralized for "Noodles": Spaghetti squash, when cooked and scraped, mimics the texture of noodles, offering a low-carb alternative.

Seasonal Abundance: Summer squashes are often abundant during the warmer months, while winter squashes are typically harvested in the fall.

Storage Longevity: Many winter squashes have a long shelf life, allowing for extended culinary enjoyment.

Ornamental Uses: Some squash varieties, especially those in the ornamental category, are used for fall decorations and centerpieces.

Conclusion:

Squash, with its diverse varieties and culinary adaptability, is a versatile and nutrient-rich addition to a well-rounded diet. Whether enjoyed as a side dish, incorporated into main courses, or used creatively in various culinary applications, squash brings both flavor and nutritional benefits to the table. As a symbol of seasonal bounty and culinary creativity, squash continues to shine in kitchens around the world.

Sweet Potatoes

Sweet potatoes, with their vibrant orange flesh and naturally sweet flavor, are not only a delicious addition to various dishes but also a nutritional powerhouse. Packed with vitamins, minerals, and fiber, sweet potatoes offer both culinary versatility and health benefits. Let's explore the characteristics, nutritional goodness, and culinary possibilities that make sweet potatoes a beloved and wholesome ingredient.

Vibrant Varieties:

- Orange-Fleshed: The most common variety, rich in beta-carotene, giving sweet potatoes their distinctive orange color.

- Purple-Fleshed: Contains anthocyanins, providing both a vibrant hue and antioxidant benefits.

- White-Fleshed: A milder flavor compared to orange sweet potatoes, with a creamy texture.

Nutrient-Rich Goodness: A one-cup (about 200 grams) serving of cooked sweet potatoes provides approximately:

- Calories: 180

- Vitamin A: 769% of the Recommended Daily Allowance (RDA)

- Vitamin C: 65% of the RDA

- Manganese: 50% of the RDA

- Fiber: 6.6 grams

Beta-Carotene and Antioxidants:

- Beta-Carotene Rich: Sweet potatoes are a potent source of beta-carotene, a precursor to vitamin A, known for its antioxidant properties.

- Anthocyanins: Purple-fleshed sweet potatoes contain anthocyanins, antioxidants associated with various health benefits.

Blood Sugar Regulation: The fiber in sweet potatoes contributes to stable blood sugar levels, making them a suitable option for individuals managing diabetes.

Heart-Healthy Potassium: Sweet potatoes contain potassium, supporting heart health by helping regulate blood pressure.

Immune System Support: Boosts the immune system and aids in collagen formation, contributing to skin health.

Culinary Versatility:

- Baked and Mashed: A classic preparation, often enhanced with a touch of cinnamon or nutmeg.

- Fries and Chips: Cut into strips or slices and baked for a healthier alternative to traditional fries.

- Soups and Stews: Added for sweetness and thickness.

- Pies and Casseroles: Featured in both sweet and savory dishes, adding depth and flavor.

- Grilled or Roasted: Enhances the natural sweetness and caramelizes the edges.

Sweet Potato Leaves: The leaves of sweet potato plants are also consumed in some cultures, providing additional nutritional benefits.

Gluten-Free and Nutrient-Dense: Sweet potatoes are a nutrient-dense option for those following gluten-free or grain-free diets.

Sustainability: Sweet potatoes are hardy and can be cultivated in diverse climates, contributing to their availability and sustainability.

Conclusion:

Sweet potatoes, with their delightful taste and nutritional richness, stand out as a wholesome and versatile food source. Whether enjoyed in classic preparations, innovative dishes, or even as nutritious alternatives to other starches, sweet potatoes continue to be a cherished ingredient in global cuisines. As a symbol of both comfort and health, sweet potatoes exemplify the harmonious combination of flavor and nutrition on the plate.

Tomatoes

Tomatoes, with their juicy and vibrant character, are not just a kitchen staple but a symbol of Mediterranean cuisine and global culinary delight. Whether consumed fresh, cooked, or processed into sauces, tomatoes bring a burst of flavor and a wealth of nutrients to a variety of dishes. Let's explore the characteristics, nutritional benefits, and culinary versatility that make tomatoes an essential and beloved ingredient.

Varied Varieties:

- Roma (Plum) Tomatoes: Oval-shaped and meaty, ideal for sauces and canning.

- Cherry Tomatoes: Small, round, and sweet, perfect for snacking and salads.

- Beefsteak Tomatoes: Large and juicy, commonly used in sandwiches and burgers.

- Heirloom Tomatoes: Unique in color, shape, and flavor, preserving historical and regional tomato varieties.

Nutrient-Rich Profile: A one-cup (about 240 grams) serving of chopped tomatoes provides approximately:

- Calories: 32

- Vitamin C: 28% of the Recommended Daily Allowance (RDA)

- Potassium: 12% of the RDA

- Vitamin K: 9% of the RDA

- Folate (Vitamin B9): 6% of the RDA

Antioxidant Lycopene: Tomatoes are rich in lycopene, an antioxidant associated with various health benefits, including heart health and cancer prevention.

Heart-Healthy Potassium: Tomatoes contribute to heart health by supporting blood pressure regulation.

Hydration and Low Calories: Tomatoes have high water content, contributing to hydration. Tomatoes are low in calories, making them a guilt-free addition to meals.

Culinary Versatility:

- Fresh in Salads: Sliced or diced tomatoes add freshness and color to salads.

- Sauces and Salsas: Cooked into rich pasta sauces, salsas, and condiments.

- Grilled and Roasted: Enhances sweetness and smokiness for a flavorful side dish.

- Stuffed Tomatoes: Hollowed tomatoes filled with various ingredients for a tasty and visually appealing dish.

- Tomato Soups: A classic comfort food, served hot or cold.

Diverse Cultural Uses:

- Mediterranean Cuisine: Integral in dishes like Caprese salad, bruschetta, and Mediterranean-style sauces.

- Latin American Cuisine: Essential in salsas, guacamole, and various sauces.

- Asian Cuisine: Used in stir-fries, curries, and pickled preparations.

Canning and Preservation: Tomatoes are commonly processed into sauces, ketchup, salsa, and canned tomatoes for year-round use.

Symbol of Summer Harvest: Tomatoes are synonymous with the summer harvest, reaching their peak in flavor and abundance.

Tomato Festivals: Some regions host tomato festivals, celebrating the fruit with events, contests, and culinary showcases.

Conclusion:

Tomatoes, with their delightful taste and nutritional richness, have earned their place as a culinary essential in kitchens worldwide. From salads to sauces, they add a burst of flavor, color, and health benefits to diverse cuisines. As a symbol of summer's bounty and a versatile ingredient, tomatoes continue to be a beloved and indispensable part of global culinary traditions.

Watercress

Watercress, with its vibrant green leaves and distinctive peppery flavor, is a nutrient-packed leafy green that has been cherished for its culinary and health benefits for centuries. Often found in salads, sandwiches, and soups, watercress not only adds a zesty kick to dishes but also offers a wealth of essential nutrients. Let's explore the characteristics, nutritional goodness, and culinary versatility that make watercress a standout among leafy greens.

Distinctive Peppery Flavor: Watercress has a bold and peppery taste, adding a zesty element to salads and various dishes.

Nutrient-Rich Profile: A one-cup (about 34 grams) serving of watercress provides approximately:

- Calories: 4

- Vitamin K: 85% of the Recommended Daily Allowance (RDA)

- Vitamin C: 14% of the RDA

- Calcium: 4% of the RDA

- Iron: 4% of the RDA

Antioxidant Power: Watercress is rich in phytonutrients, including beta-carotene and flavonoids, contributing to its antioxidant properties.

Bone Health Support: Essential for bone health, vitamin K plays a role in bone mineralization and density.

Immune System Boost: Supports the immune system, helps in collagen formation, and acts as an antioxidant.

Digestive Health: Watercress provides dietary fiber, promoting digestive health and contributing to regular bowel movements.

Culinary Versatility:

- Fresh in Salads: Enjoyed as a base or addition to salads, providing a peppery kick.

- Sandwiches and Wraps: Adds crunch and flavor to sandwiches and wraps.

- Soups and Stews: Used in hot dishes, adding a burst of freshness and nutrients.

- Pesto: Watercress can be used as a peppery alternative to basil in pesto recipes.

Watercress Smoothies: Watercress can be blended into smoothies for a nutrient boost, contributing a unique flavor.

Historical Medicinal Use: Historically, watercress has been used in traditional medicine for various purposes, including as a digestive aid and a source of vitamins.

Aquatic Growth Habit: Watercress often grows near clean, flowing water, absorbing nutrients from the water, which contributes to its nutrient density.

Conclusion:

Watercress, with its peppery flavor and nutrient-rich profile, stands out as a versatile and healthful leafy green. Whether enjoyed in salads, soups, or blended into smoothies, watercress adds a unique zing and nutritional goodness to culinary creations. As a symbol of freshness and vitality, watercress continues to be a celebrated ingredient in the world of leafy greens, contributing both flavor and essential nutrients to a balanced and vibrant diet.

Watermelon

Watermelon, with its vibrant pink flesh and unmistakable sweetness, is a quintessential summer fruit cherished for its hydrating properties and delicious taste. Comprising mostly water, watermelon is not only a refreshing treat but also offers a range of essential nutrients. Let's explore the characteristics, nutritional benefits, and the sheer delight that watermelon brings to summertime.

Juicy and Hydrating: Watermelon is composed of over 90% water, making it a perfect choice for staying hydrated, especially during hot summer days.

Nutrient-Rich Goodness: A one-cup (about 152 grams) serving of watermelon provides approximately:

- Calories: 46

- Vitamin C: 21% of the Recommended Daily Allowance (RDA)

- Vitamin A: 18% of the RDA

- Potassium: 5% of the RDA

Antioxidant Lycopene: Watermelon is a rich source of lycopene, an antioxidant associated with various health benefits, including heart health.

Hydration and Electrolytes: Contains electrolytes like potassium, which aids in fluid balance and muscle function.

Low in Calories: With its low-calorie content, watermelon is a guilt-free and satisfying snack.

Cooling and Refreshing: Watermelon's natural sweetness and high water content make it a popular choice for cooling down and satisfying sweet cravings during the summer.

Culinary Versatility:

- Sliced and Diced: Enjoyed fresh, either sliced or diced, for a quick and hydrating snack.

- Salads and Salsas: Added to fruit salads, tossed salads, or salsas for a burst of color and sweetness.

- Smoothies and Beverages: Blended into refreshing smoothies, juices, or cocktails.

- Frozen Treats: Favored in frozen treats like watermelon popsicles or granitas.

Seedless Varieties: Seedless watermelon varieties reduce the hassle of dealing with seeds, enhancing the overall eating experience.

Symbol of Summer Celebrations: Watermelon is a classic addition to outdoor gatherings, picnics, and barbecues, symbolizing summer celebrations.

Sustainable and Edible Rind: The rind, often discarded, is edible and can be pickled or used in creative recipes, contributing to sustainable food practices.

Conclusion:

Watermelon, with its hydrating nature, vibrant color, and delightful taste, embodies the essence of summer. Whether enjoyed in its pure form, incorporated into dishes, or transformed into frozen treats, watermelon is a versatile and healthful addition to the summer menu. As a symbol of seasonal joy and refreshment, watermelon continues to be a favorite among people of all ages during the warmer months.

Zucchini

Zucchini, a member of the squash family, is a versatile and mild-flavored vegetable that adds both nutritional value and culinary flair to a variety of dishes. With its tender texture and mild taste, zucchini can be prepared in numerous ways, making it a favorite among home cooks and chefs alike. Let's explore the characteristics, nutritional benefits, and culinary versatility that make zucchini a popular and delightful addition to meals.

Mild Flavor and Tender Texture:

- Neutral Taste: Zucchini has a mild, almost neutral flavor, making it adaptable to various culinary preparations.

- Tender Texture: The tender flesh of zucchini lends itself well to both quick cooking and longer, slow-cooked dishes.

Nutrient-Rich Goodness: A one-cup (about 180 grams) serving of sliced, cooked zucchini provides approximately:

- Calories: 20

- Vitamin C: 36% of the Recommended Daily Allowance (RDA)

- Vitamin A: 10% of the RDA

- Potassium: 8% of the RDA

- Fiber: 2 grams

Low in Calories and Carbs:

- Calorie-Friendly: Zucchini is a low-calorie vegetable, making it a suitable choice for those watching their calorie intake.

- Low Carbohydrates: With a low carbohydrate content, zucchini is often included in low-carb and keto-friendly diets.

Antioxidant Content: Zucchini contains antioxidants like lutein and zeaxanthin, which are beneficial for eye health.

Hydration and Dietary Fiber:

- Water Content: Zucchini has a high water content, contributing to hydration.

- Dietary Fiber: The fiber in zucchini supports digestive health and promotes a feeling of fullness.

Culinary Versatility:

- Sautéed and Stir-Fried: Quickly cooked with herbs and spices for a simple and flavorful side dish.

- Grilled and Roasted: Enhances sweetness and adds a smoky flavor when grilled or roasted.

- Spiralized for "Zoodles": Spiralized zucchini can be used as a low-carb alternative to noodles in various dishes.

- Baked in Casseroles: Incorporated into casseroles, lasagnas, or gratins for added texture and nutrition.

Garden-to-Table Appeal: Zucchini is a popular choice among home gardeners for its ease of cultivation and prolific harvest.

Stuffed Zucchini: Zucchini can be hollowed and stuffed with a variety of ingredients like cheese, grains, or proteins.

Sweet Zucchini Breads: Zucchini is often used in baking, adding moisture and nutrition to sweet treats like zucchini bread or muffins.

Seasonal Bounty: Zucchini is abundant during the summer months, offering a fresh and seasonal ingredient to meals.

Conclusion:

Zucchini, with its versatility and nutritional benefits, stands out as a culinary gem in the world of vegetables. Whether enjoyed as a simple side dish, a creative main course, or a delightful baked treat, zucchini adds both flavor and nutrition to a variety of dishes. As a symbol of garden abundance and culinary creativity, zucchini continues to be a cherished ingredient on plates around the world.

www.ingramcontent.com/pod-product-compliance
Lightning Source LLC
Chambersburg PA
CBHW070911260726

48661CB00004B/1692